Gerontological Social Work and COVID-19

The novel coronavirus and the resultant COVID-19 pandemic have disproportionately affected older adults in terms of the number of lives lost, concerns about the safety of institutional and home and community-based care, the impact of isolation and seclusion, and the ability to participate and engage in meaningful and contributory activities. The pandemic has uncovered layers of ageism that are embedded in societies globally and challenges us all to address the pervasive individual, institutional, and structural biases that permit age-based discrimination. Within the interdisciplinary field of gerontology, social workers lead organizations, provide direct services and supports, facilitate community engagement and participation, and deliver therapeutic interventions among other roles and activities that facilitate positive outcomes for older adults and their families.

In *Gerontological Social Work and COVID-19: Calls for Change in Education, Practice, and Policy from International Voices*, scholars, practice professionals, and other stakeholders reflect on the initial months of the pandemic. They articulate immediate needs the pandemic has created and uncovered, and further identify directions the field must go in to meet the moment and prepare for the future ahead.

This book was originally published as a special issue of the *Journal of Gerontological Social Work*.

Michelle Putnam, PhD, is Professor and Director of the PhD Program at the School of Social Work, College of Social Sciences, Policy, and Practice, Simmons University in Boston, USA. She is the Editor-in-Chief of the *Journal of Gerontological Social Work*.

Huei-Wern Shen, PhD, is Associate Professor in the Department of Social Work, College of Health and Public Service, University of North Texas in Denton, USA. She is the Managing Editor of the *Journal of Gerontological Social Work*.

Gerontological Social Work and COVID-19

Calls for Change in Education, Practice, and Policy from International Voices

Edited by
Michelle Putnam and Huei-Wern Shen

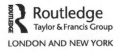

Routledge
Taylor & Francis Group

LONDON AND NEW YORK

First published 2022
by Routledge
2 Park Square, Milton Park, Abingdon, Oxon, OX14 4RN

and by Routledge
605 Third Avenue, New York, NY 10158

Routledge is an imprint of the Taylor & Francis Group, an informa business

British Library Cataloguing-in-Publication Data
A catalogue record for this book is available from the British Library

ISBN13: 978-0-367-68610-9 (hbk)
ISBN13: 978-0-367-68613-0 (pbk)
ISBN13: 978-1-003-13828-0 (ebk)

DOI: 10.4324/9781003138280

Typeset in Minion Pro
by codeMantra

Publisher's Note
The publisher accepts responsibility for any inconsistencies that may have arisen during the conversion of this book from journal articles to book chapters, namely the inclusion of journal terminology.

Disclaimer
Every effort has been made to contact copyright holders for their permission to reprint material in this book. The publishers would be grateful to hear from any copyright holder who is not here acknowledged and will undertake to rectify any errors or omissions in future editions of this book.

Contents

Citation Information   xi
Notes on Contributors   xviii

Introduction   1
Michelle Putnam and Huei-Wern Shen

PART I
Commentaries on Gerontological Social Work's Response to COVID-19   7

1 The Consequences of Ageist Language are upon us   9
   Clara Berridge and Nancy Hooyman

2 Applying Gerontological Social Work Perspectives to the Coronavirus Pandemic 14
   Emma Swinford, Natalie Galucia, and Nancy Morrow-Howell

3 COVID-19 Pandemic: Workforce Implications for Gerontological Social Work   25
   Marla Berg-Weger and Tracy Schroepfer

4 Older Workers in the Time of COVID-19: The Senior Community Service
   Employment Program and Implications for Social Work   31
   Cal J. Halvorsen and Olga Yulikova

5 Caregiving in Times of Uncertainty: Helping Adult Children of Aging
   Parents Find Support during the COVID-19 Outbreak   43
   Elizabeth Lightfoot and Rajean P. Moone

PART II
Gerontological Social Work Role in Addressing COVID-19   55

6 Gerontological Social Work's Pivotal Role in the COVID-19 Pandemic:
   A Response from AGESW Leadership   57
   Tam E. Perry, Nancy Kusmaul, and Cal J. Halvorsen

7   The Impact of the COVID-19 Pandemic on Vulnerable Older Adults in the
    United States   63
    Yeonjung Jane Lee

8   Social Work Values in Action during COVID-19   69
    Vivian J. Miller and HeeSoon Lee

9   COVID-19 and Older Adults: The Time for Gerontology-Curriculum across
    Social Work Programs is Now!   74
    Susanny J. Beltran and Vivian J. Miller

10 They are Essential Workers Now, and Should
    Continue to Be: Social Workers and Home Health Care Workers during
    COVID-19 and Beyond   78
    *Lourdes R. Guerrero, Ariel C. Avgar, Erica Phillips,
    and Madeline R. Sterling*

11 A Reflection of and Charge to Gerontological Social Work: Past Pandemics
    and the Current COVID-19 Crisis   81
    Tyrone C. Hamler, Sara J. English, Susanny J. Beltran, and Vivian J. Miller

PART III
COVID-19 and Social Work with Diverse Groups   **85**

12 The Disproportionate Impact of COVID-19 on Minority Groups: A Social
    Justice Concern   87
    HeeSoon Lee and Vivian J. Miller

13 Social Workers Must Address Intersecting Vulnerabilities among
    Noninstitutionalized, Black, Latinx, and Older Adults of Color during the
    COVID-19 Pandemic   92
    Megan T. Ebor, Tamra B. Loeb, and Laura Trejo

14 Expanding Bilingual Social Workers for the East Asian Older Adults
    beyond the "COVID-19 Racism"   96
    Sangeun Lee

15 Older Latinx Immigrants and Covid-19: A Call to Action   99
    Rocío Calvo

16 Social Work Response Needed to the Challenge of COVID-19 for Aging
    People with Intellectual and Developmental Disabilties   102
    Philip McCallion

17 Unraveling the Invisible but Harmful Impact of COVID-19 on Deaf Older
    Adults and Older Adults with Hearing Loss   105
    Junghyun Park

18 The Impact of COVID-19 on Older Adults Living with HIV: HIV Care and
    Psychosocial Effects   109
    Monique J. Brown and Sharon B. Weissman

19 Serving LGBTQ+/SGL Elders during the Novel Corona Virus (COVID-19)
    Pandemic: Striving for Justice, Recognizing Resilience   114
    Sarah Jen, Dan Stewart, and Imani Woody

20 Older Adults and Covid 19: Social Justice, Disparities, and
    Social Work Practice   118
    Carole Cox

PART IV
COVID-19 and Health and Social Care   **133**

21 Self-Direction of Home and Community-Based Services in the
    Time of COVID-19   135
    Kevin J. Mahoney

22 COVID-19 Pandemic: Opportunity to Advanced Home
    Care for Older Adults   139
    Vahidreza Borhaninejad and Vahid Rashedi

23 The Need for Community Practice to Support Aging in Place during COVID-19 141
    Althea Pestine-Stevens and Emily A. Greenfield

24 Covid-19 and Community Care in South Korea   145
    Soyoon Weon

25 Social Work with Older Persons Living with Dementia in Nigeria: COVID-19 148
    Oluwagbemiga Oyinlola and Oluromade Olusa

26 Thoughts on Living in a Nursing Facility during the Pandemic   152
    Penny Shaw

27 The Care Home Pandemic – What Lessons Can We Learn for the Future?   154
    Ameer A. Khan, Vineshwar P. Singh, and Darab Khan

28 Nursing Home in the COVID-19 Outbreak: Challenge, Recovery,
    and Resiliency   156
    *Huanhuan Huang, Yan Xie, Zhiyu Chen, Mingzhao Xiao, Songmei Cao,
    Jie Mi, Xiuli Yu, and Qinghua Zhao*

29 Nursing Home Social Work During COVID-19   161
    *Nancy Kusmaul, Mercedes Bern-Klug, Jennifer Heston-Mullins, Amy R.
    Roberts, and Colleen Galambos*

30 Working with Older Caregivers of Persons with Mental Illness during
    COVID-19: Decreasing Burden, Creating Plans for Future Care, and
    Utilizing Strengths   164
    Travis Labrum, Christina Newhill, and Tyler Smathers

31 Service Needs of Older Adults with Serious Mental Illness   169
    Nathaniel A. Dell, Natsuki Sasaki, Madeline Stewart, Allison M. Murphy,
    and Marina Klier

32 The Implications of COVID-19 for the Mental Health Care of Older Adults:
    Insights from Emergency Department Social Workers   172
    Xiaoling Xiang, Yawen Ning, and Jay Kayser

33 Psychosocial Impact of COVID-19 on Older Adults: A Cultural Geriatric
    Mental Health- Care Perspectived   175
    Sonia Mukhtar

PART V
Social Isolation and the Digital Experience in COVID-19   **179**

34 Practical Implications of Physical Distancing, Social Isolation, and Reduced
    Physicality for Older Adults in Response to COVID-19   181
    Anthony D. Campbell

35 COVID-19 and the Digital Divide: Will Social Workers Help
    Bridge the Gap?   184
    Allison Gibson, Shoshana H. Bardach, and Natalie D. Pope

36 The Digital Exclusion of Older Adults during the COVID-19 Pandemic   187
    Alexander Seifert

37 Choosing Physical Distancing over Social Distancing in the Era of
    Technology: Minimizing Risk for Older People   190
    Saptarshi Chatterjee

38 Virtual Social Work Care with Older Black Adults: A Culturally Relevant
    Technology-Based Intervention to Reduce Social Isolation and Loneliness in
    a Time of Pandemic   192
    Sulaimon Giwa, Delores V. Mullings, and Karun K. Karki

39 Social Responses for Older People in COVID-19 Pandemic:
    Experience from Vietnam   195
    Le Thanh Tung

40 Fighting COVID-19: Fear and Internal Conflict among Older
    Adults in Ghana   201
    Razak M Gyasi

41 Re-integrating Older Adults Who Have Recovered from the Novel
   Coronavirus into Society in the Context of Stigmatization: Lessons for
   Health and Social Actors in Ghana   204
   Williams Agyemang-Duah, Anthony Kwame Morgan, Joseph Oduro Appiah,
   Prince Peprah, and Audrey Amponsah Fordjour

PART VI
Interventions to Support Older Adults during COVID-19   **207**

42 Staying Isolated in Order to Stay Safe: Exploring Experiences of the MIT
   AgeLab 85+ Lifestyle Leaders during the COVID-19 Pandemic   209
   Julie B. Miller, Taylor R. Patskanick, Lisa A. D'Ambrosio, and Joseph F. Coughlin

43 Adapting 'Sunshine,' A Socially Assistive Chat Robot for Older Adults with
   Cognitive Impairment: A Pilot Study   211
   Othelia EunKyoung Lee and Boyd Davis

44 Reaching older adults during the COVID-19 pandemic through social
   networks and Social Security Schemes in Ghana: Lessons for considerations 214
   Francis Arthur-Holmes and Williams Agyemang-Duah

45 Animal (Non-human) Companionship for Adults Aging in Place during
   COVID-19: A Critical Support, a Source of Concern and Potential for Social
   Work Responses   217
   Mary E. Rauktis and Janet Hoy-Gerlach

46 Detroit's Efforts to Meet the Needs of Seniors: Macro Responses to a Crisis 221
   Dennis Archambault, Claudia Sanford, and Tam Perry

47 Foregrounding Context in the COVID-19 Pandemic: Learning from Older
   Adults in Puerto Rico   224
   Denise Burnette, Tommy D. Buckley, Humberto E. Fabelo, and Mauricio P. Yabar

48 An Innovative Telephone Outreach Program to Seniors in Detroit, a City
   Facing Dire Consequences of COVID-19   228
   Vanessa Rorai and Tam E. Perry

49 Healthcare Concerns of Older Adults during the COVID-19 Outbreak in
   Low- and Middle- Income Countries: Lessons for Health Policy
   and Social Work   232
   Francis Arthur-Holmes, Michael Kwesi Asare Akaadom, Williams
   Agyemang-Duah, Kwaku Abrefa Busia, and Prince Peprah

50 Geriatric Health in Bangladesh during COVID-19: Challenges
   and Recommendations   239
   Md Mahbub Hossain, Hoimonty Mazumder, Samia Tasnim, Tasmiah
   Nuzhath, and Abida Sultana

51 Lessons for Averting the Delayed and Reduced Patronage of non-COVID-19
    Medical Services by Older People in Ghana   243
    Anthony Kwame Morgan and Beatrice Aberinpoka Awafo

    Index   247

Citation Information

The chapters in this book were originally published in the *Journal of Gerontological Social Work*, volume 63, issue 6–7 (2020). When citing this material, please use the original page numbering for each article, as follows:

Introduction
Gerontological Social Work and COVID-19: Calls for Change in Education, Practice, and Policy from International Voices
Michelle Putnam and Huei-Wern Shen
Journal of Gerontological Social Work, volume 63, issue 6–7 (2020) pp. 503–507

Chapter 1
The Consequences of Ageist Language are upon us
Clara Berridge and Nancy Hooyman
Journal of Gerontological Social Work, volume 63, issue 6–7 (2020) pp. 508–512

Chapter 2
Applying Gerontological Social Work Perspectives to the Coronavirus Pandemic
Emma Swinford, Natalie Galucia, and Nancy Morrow-Howell
Journal of Gerontological Social Work, volume 63, issue 6–7 (2020) pp. 513–523

Chapter 3
COVID-19 Pandemic: Workforce Implications for Gerontological Social Work
Marla Berg-Weger and Tracy Schroepfer
Journal of Gerontological Social Work, volume 63, issue 6–7 (2020) pp. 524–529

Chapter 4
Older Workers in the Time of COVID-19: The Senior Community Service Employment Program and Implications for Social Work
Cal J. Halvorsen and Olga Yulikova
Journal of Gerontological Social Work, volume 63, issue 6–7 (2020) pp. 530–541

Chapter 5
Caregiving in Times of Uncertainty: Helping Adult Children of Aging Parents Find Support during the COVID-19 Outbreak
Elizabeth Lightfoot and Rajean P. Moone
Journal of Gerontological Social Work, volume 63, issue 6–7 (2020) pp. 542–552

Chapter 6

Gerontological Social Work's Pivotal Role in the COVID-19 Pandemic: A Response from AGESW Leadership

Tam E. Perry, Nancy Kusmaul, and Cal J. Halvorsen

Journal of Gerontological Social Work, volume 63, issue 6–7 (2020) pp. 553–558

Chapter 7

The Impact of the COVID-19 Pandemic on Vulnerable Older Adults in the United States

Yeonjung Jane Lee

Journal of Gerontological Social Work, volume 63, issue 6–7 (2020) pp. 559–564

Chapter 8

Social Work Values in Action during COVID-19

Vivian J. Miller and HeeSoon Lee

Journal of Gerontological Social Work, volume 63, issue 6–7 (2020) pp. 565–569

Chapter 9

COVID-19 and Older Adults: The Time for Gerontology-Curriculum across Social Work Programs is Now!

Susanny J. Beltran and Vivian J. Miller

Journal of Gerontological Social Work, volume 63, issue 6–7 (2020) pp. 570–573

Chapter 10

They are Essential Workers Now, and Should Continue to Be: Social Workers and Home Health Care Workers during COVID-19 and Beyond

Lourdes R. Guerrero, Ariel C. Avgar, Erica Phillips, and Madeline R. Sterling

Journal of Gerontological Social Work, volume 63, issue 6–7 (2020) pp. 574–576

Chapter 11

A Reflection of and Charge to Gerontological Social Work: Past Pandemics and the Current COVID-19 Crisis

Tyrone C. Hamler, Sara J. English, Susanny J. Beltran, and Vivian J. Miller

Journal of Gerontological Social Work, volume 63, issue 6–7 (2020) pp. 577–579

Chapter 12

The Disproportionate Impact of COVID-19 on Minority Groups: A Social Justice Concern

HeeSoon Lee and Vivian J. Miller

Journal of Gerontological Social Work, volume 63, issue 6–7 (2020) pp. 580–584

Chapter 13

Social Workers Must Address Intersecting Vulnerabilities among Noninstitutionalized, Black, Latinx, and Older Adults of Color during the COVID-19 Pandemic

Megan T. Ebor, Tamra B. Loeb, and Laura Trejo

Journal of Gerontological Social Work, volume 63, issue 6–7 (2020) pp. 585–588

Chapter 14

Expanding Bilingual Social Workers for the East Asian Older Adults beyond the "COVID-19 Racism"

Sangeun Lee

Journal of Gerontological Social Work, volume 63, issue 6–7 (2020) pp. 589–591

Chapter 15

Older Latinx Immigrants and Covid-19: A Call to Action

Rocío Calvo

Journal of Gerontological Social Work, volume 63, issue 6–7 (2020) pp. 592–594

Chapter 16

Social Work Response Needed to the Challenge of COVID-19 for Aging People with Intellectual and Developmental Disabilties

Philip McCallion

Journal of Gerontological Social Work, volume 63, issue 6–7 (2020) pp. 595–597

Chapter 17

Unraveling the Invisible but Harmful Impact of COVID-19 on Deaf Older Adults and Older Adults with Hearing Loss

Junghyun Park

Journal of Gerontological Social Work, volume 63, issue 6–7 (2020) pp. 598–601

Chapter 18

The Impact of COVID-19 on Older Adults Living with HIV: HIV Care and Psychosocial Effects

Monique J. Brown and Sharon B. Weissman

Journal of Gerontological Social Work, volume 63, issue 6–7 (2020) pp. 602–606

Chapter 19

Serving LGBTQ+/SGL Elders during the Novel Corona Virus (COVID-19) Pandemic: Striving for Justice, Recognizing Resilience

Sarah Jen, Dan Stewart, and Imani Woody

Journal of Gerontological Social Work, volume 63, issue 6–7 (2020) pp. 607–610

Chapter 20

Older Adults and Covid 19: Social Justice, Disparities, and Social Work Practice

Carole Cox

Journal of Gerontological Social Work, volume 63, issue 6–7 (2020) pp. 611–624

Chapter 21

Self-Direction of Home and Community-Based Services in the Time of COVID-19

Kevin J. Mahoney

Journal of Gerontological Social Work, volume 63, issue 6–7 (2020) pp. 625–628

Chapter 22

COVID-19 Pandemic: Opportunity to Advanced Home Care for Older Adults
Vahidreza Borhaninejad and Vahid Rashedi
Journal of Gerontological Social Work, volume 63, issue 6–7 (2020) pp. 629–630

Chapter 23

The Need for Community Practice to Support Aging in Place during COVID-19
Althea Pestine-Stevens and Emily A. Greenfield
Journal of Gerontological Social Work, volume 63, issue 6–7 (2020) pp. 631–634

Chapter 24

Covid-19 and Community Care in South Korea
Soyoon Weon
Journal of Gerontological Social Work, volume 63, issue 6–7 (2020) pp. 635–637

Chapter 25

Social Work with Older Persons Living with Dementia in Nigeria: COVID-19
Oluwagbemiga Oyinlola and Oluromade Olusa
Journal of Gerontological Social Work, volume 63, issue 6–7 (2020) pp. 638–641

Chapter 26

Thoughts on Living in a Nursing Facility during the Pandemic
Penny Shaw
Journal of Gerontological Social Work, volume 63, issue 6–7 (2020) pp. 642–643

Chapter 27

The Care Home Pandemic – What Lessons Can We Learn for the Future?
Ameer A. Khan, Vineshwar P. Singh, and Darab Khan
Journal of Gerontological Social Work, volume 63, issue 6–7 (2020) pp. 644–645

Chapter 28

Nursing Home in the COVID-19 Outbreak: Challenge, Recovery, and Resiliency
Huanhuan Huang, Yan Xie, Zhiyu Chen, Mingzhao Xiao, Songmei Cao, Jie Mi, Xiuli Yu, and Qinghua Zhao
Journal of Gerontological Social Work, volume 63, issue 6–7 (2020) pp. 646–650

Chapter 29

Nursing Home Social Work During COVID-19
Nancy Kusmaul, Mercedes Bern-Klug, Jennifer Heston-Mullins, Amy R. Roberts, and Colleen Galambos
Journal of Gerontological Social Work, volume 63, issue 6–7 (2020) pp. 651–653

Chapter 30

Working with Older Caregivers of Persons with Mental Illness during COVID-19: Decreasing Burden, Creating Plans for Future Care, and Utilizing Strengths
Travis Labrum, Christina Newhill, and Tyler Smathers
Journal of Gerontological Social Work, volume 63, issue 6–7 (2020) pp. 654–658

Chapter 31
Service Needs of Older Adults with Serious Mental Illness
Nathaniel A. Dell, Natsuki Sasaki, Madeline Stewart, Allison M. Murphy, and Marina Klier
Journal of Gerontological Social Work, volume 63, issue 6–7 (2020) pp. 659–661

Chapter 32
The Implications of COVID-19 for the Mental Health Care of Older Adults: Insights from Emergency Department Social Workers
Xiaoling Xiang, Yawen Ning, and Jay Kayser
Journal of Gerontological Social Work, volume 63, issue 6–7 (2020) pp. 662–664

Chapter 33
Psychosocial Impact of COVID-19 on Older Adults: A Cultural Geriatric Mental Health-Care Perspectived
Sonia Mukhtar
Journal of Gerontological Social Work, volume 63, issue 6–7 (2020) pp. 665–667

Chapter 34
Practical Implications of Physical Distancing, Social Isolation, and Reduced Physicality for Older Adults in Response to COVID-19
Anthony D. Campbell
Journal of Gerontological Social Work, volume 63, issue 6–7 (2020) pp. 668–670

Chapter 35
COVID-19 and the Digital Divide: Will Social Workers Help Bridge the Gap?
Allison Gibson, Shoshana H. Bardach, and Natalie D. Pope
Journal of Gerontological Social Work, volume 63, issue 6–7 (2020) pp. 671–673

Chapter 36
The Digital Exclusion of Older Adults during the COVID-19 Pandemic
Alexander Seifert
Journal of Gerontological Social Work, volume 63, issue 6–7 (2020) pp. 674–676

Chapter 37
Choosing Physical Distancing over Social Distancing in the Era of Technology: Minimizing Risk for Older People
Saptarshi Chatterjee
Journal of Gerontological Social Work, volume 63, issue 6–7 (2020) pp. 677–678

Chapter 38
Virtual Social Work Care with Older Black Adults: A Culturally Relevant Technology-Based Intervention to Reduce Social Isolation and Loneliness in a Time of Pandemic
Sulaimon Giwa, Delores V. Mullings, and Karun K. Karki
Journal of Gerontological Social Work, volume 63, issue 6–7 (2020) pp. 679–681

Chapter 39

Social Responses for Older People in COVID-19 Pandemic: Experience from Vietnam
Le Thanh Tung
Journal of Gerontological Social Work, volume 63, issue 6–7 (2020) pp. 682–687

Chapter 40

Fighting COVID-19: Fear and Internal Conflict among Older Adults in Ghana
Razak M Gyasi
Journal of Gerontological Social Work, volume 63, issue 6–7 (2020) pp. 688–690

Chapter 41

*Re-integrating Older Adults Who Have Recovered from the Novel Coronavirus into Society
in the Context of Stigmatization: Lessons for Health and Social Actors in Ghana*
Williams Agyemang-Duah, Anthony Kwame Morgan, Joseph Oduro Appiah, Prince
Peprah, and Audrey Amponsah Fordjour
Journal of Gerontological Social Work, volume 63, issue 6–7 (2020) pp. 691–693

Chapter 42

*Staying Isolated in Order to Stay Safe: Exploring Experiences of the MIT AgeLab 85+ Life-
style Leaders during the COVID-19 Pandemic*
Julie B. Miller, Taylor R. Patskanick, Lisa A. D'Ambrosio, and Joseph F. Coughlin
Journal of Gerontological Social Work, volume 63, issue 6–7 (2020) pp. 694–695

Chapter 43

*Adapting 'Sunshine,' A Socially Assistive Chat Robot for Older Adults with Cognitive Im-
pairment: A Pilot Study*
Othelia EunKyoung Lee and Boyd Davis
Journal of Gerontological Social Work, volume 63, issue 6–7 (2020) pp. 520–528

Chapter 44

*Reaching older adults during the COVID-19 pandemic through social networks and Social
Security Schemes in Ghana: Lessons for considerations*
Francis Arthur-Holmes and Williams Agyemang-Duah
Journal of Gerontological Social Work, volume 63, issue 6–7 (2020) pp. 699–701

Chapter 45

*Animal (Non-human) Companionship for Adults Aging in Place during COVID-19: A Crit-
ical Support, a Source of Concern and Potential for Social Work Responses*
Mary E. Rauktis and Janet Hoy-Gerlach
Journal of Gerontological Social Work, volume 63, issue 6–7 (2020) pp. 702–705

Chapter 46

Detroit's Efforts to Meet the Needs of Seniors: Macro Responses to a Crisis
Dennis Archambault, Claudia Sanford, and Tam Perry
Journal of Gerontological Social Work, volume 63, issue 6–7 (2020) pp. 520–528

Chapter 47

Foregrounding Context in the COVID-19 Pandemic: Learning from Older Adults in Puerto Rico

Denise Burnette, Tommy D. Buckley, Humberto E. Fabelo, and Mauricio P. Yabar

Journal of Gerontological Social Work, volume 63, issue 6–7 (2020) pp. 709–712

Chapter 48

An Innovative Telephone Outreach Program to Seniors in Detroit, a City Facing Dire Consequences of COVID-19

Vanessa Rorai and Tam E. Perry

Journal of Gerontological Social Work, volume 63, issue 6–7 (2020) pp. 713–716

Chapter 49

Healthcare Concerns of Older Adults during the COVID-19 Outbreak in Low- and Middle-Income Countries: Lessons for Health Policy and Social Work

Francis Arthur-Holmes, Michael Kwesi Asare Akaadom, Williams Agyemang-Duah, Kwaku Abrefa Busia, and Prince Peprah

Journal of Gerontological Social Work, volume 63, issue 6–7 (2020) pp. 717–723

Chapter 50

Geriatric Health in Bangladesh during COVID-19: Challenges and Recommendations

Md Mahbub Hossain, Hoimonty Mazumder, Samia Tasnim, Tasmiah Nuzhath, and Abida Sultana

Journal of Gerontological Social Work, volume 63, issue 6–7 (2020) pp. 724–727

Chapter 51

Lessons for Averting the Delayed and Reduced Patronage of non-COVID-19 Medical Services by Older People in Ghana

Anthony Kwame Morgan and Beatrice Aberinpoka Awafo

Journal of Gerontological Social Work, volume 63, issue 6–7 (2020) pp. 728–731

For any permission-related enquiries please visit:
http://www.tandfonline.com/page/help/permissions

Contributors

Williams Agyemang-Duah Department of Planning, Kwame Nkrumah University of Science and Technology, Kumasi, Ghana.

Michael Kwesi Asare Akaadom School of Pharmacy, Central University, Accra, Ghana.

Audrey Amponsah Fordjour Cape Breton Regional Hospital, Sydney, Canada.

Joseph Oduro Appiah University of Northern British Columbia, Prince George, Canada.

Dennis Archambault Authority Health & Communications. Senior Housing Preservation-Detroit, USA.

Francis Arthur-Holmes Oxford Department of International Development, University of Oxford, England, UK.

Ariel C. Avgar Cornell University, Ithaca, New York, USA.

Beatrice Aberinpoka Awafo Department of Geography and Rural Development, Kwame Nkrumah University of Science and Technology (KNUST), Kumasi, Ghana.

Shoshana H. Bardach University of Kentucky Department of Gerontology, Lexington, USA.

Susanny J. Beltran School of Social Work, University of Central Florida, Orlando, USA.

Marla Berg-Weger School of Social Work and Gateway Geriatric Education Center, Saint Louis University, St. Louis, USA.

Mercedes Bern-Klug School of Social Work, University of Iowa, USA.

Clara Berridge School of Social Work, University of Washington, Seattle, USA.

Vahidreza Borhaninejad Social Determinants of Health Research Center, Institute for Futures Studies in Health, Kerman University of Medical Sciences, Iran.

Monique J. Brown Department of Epidemiology and Biostatistics, Arnold School of Public Health, University of South Carolina, Columbia, USA.

Sharon B. Weissman Department of Internal Medicine, School of Medicine, University of South Carolina, Columbia, USA.

Tommy D. Buckley Virginia Commonwealth University School of Social Work, Academic Learning Commons, Richmond, USA.

Denise Burnette Virginia Commonwealth University School of Social Work, Academic Learning Commons, Richmond, USA.

Kwaku Abrefa Busia Department of Sociology and Social Policy, Lingnan University, Tuen Mun, New Territories, Hong Kong.

Rocío Calvo Boston College School of Social Work, McGuinn Hall, MA.

Anthony D. Campbell Department of Sociology, Anthropology, and Social Work, Auburn University, Auburn, USA.

Songmei Cao Department of Nursing, The First Affiliated Hospital of Chongqing Medical University, China.

Saptarshi Chatterjee Department of Microbiology, Adamas University, Kolkata, India.

Zhiyu Chen Department of Orthopaedic, The First Affiliated Hospital of Chongqing Medical University, China.

Joseph F. Coughlin AgeLab, Massachusetts Institute of Technology, Cambridge, USA.

Carole Cox Graduate School of Social Service, Fordham University, New York, USA.

Lisa A. D'Ambrosio AgeLab, Massachusetts Institute of Technology, Cambridge, USA.

Boyd Davis The University of North Carolina, Charlotte, USA.

Nathaniel A. Dell Places for People, Inc., Saint Louis, USA.

Megan T. Ebor Department of Psychiatry and Biobehavioral Sciences, University of California, USA.

Sara J. English Department of Social Work, Winthrop University, Rock Hill, USA.

Humberto E. Fabelo Virginia Commonwealth University School of Social Work, Academic Learning Commons, Richmond, USA.

Colleen Galambos University of Wisconsin Milwaukee, USA.

Natalie Galucia Harvey A. Friedman Center for Aging, Washington University, St. Louis, USA.

Allison Gibson Assistant Professor, University of Kentucky College of Social Work, Lexington, USA.

Sulaimon Giwa School of Social Work, Memorial University of Newfoundland, St. John's, Canada.

Emily A. Greenfield School of Social Work, Rutgers, The State University of New Jersey, New Brunswick, USA.

Lourdes R. Guerrero Division of Geriatrics, Department of Medicine, David Geffen School of Medicine at UCLA, Los Angeles, USA.

Razak M Gyasi Aging and Development Unit, African Population and Health Research Center (APHRC), Nairobi, Kenya.

Cal J. Halvorsen Boston College School of Social Work, Chestnut Hill, USA.

Tyrone C. Hamler Case Western Reserve University, Cleveland, USA.

Jennifer Heston-Mullins Scripps Gerontology Center, Miami University, Oxford, USA.

Nancy Hooyman School of Social Work, University of Washington, Seattle, USA.

Md Mahbub Hossain Department of Health Promotion and Community Health Sciences, Texas A&M School of Public Health, College Station, USA.

Janet Hoy-Gerlach Social Work Program, The University of Toledo, USA.

Huanhuan Huang Department of Nursing, The First Affiliated Hospital of Chongqing Medical University, China.

Sarah Jen School of Social Welfare, University of Kansas, Lawrence, USA.

Karun K. Karki School of Social Work and Human Services, University of the Fraser Valley, Abbotsford, Canada.

Jay Kayser Departments of Social Work and Developmental Psychology, University of Michigan, Ann Arbor, USA.

Ameer A. Khan School of Medicine, University of Liverpool, England, UK.

Darab Khan School of Medicine, University of Liverpool, England, UK.

Marina Klier Places for People, Inc., Saint Louis, USA.

Nancy Kusmaul Department of Social Work, University of Maryland Baltimore County, USA.

Travis Labrum School of Social Work, University of Pittsburgh, USA.

Othelia EunKyoung Lee The University of North Carolina, Charlotte, USA.

Yeonjung Jane Lee Myron B. Thompson School of Social Work, University of Hawai'i at Mānoa, Honolulu, USA.

HeeSoon Lee Department of Human Services, Bowling Green State University, USA.

Sangeun Lee Graduate School of Social Work and Social Research, Bryn Mawr College, USA.

Elizabeth Lightfoot School of Social Work, University of Minnesota, USA.

Tamra B. Loeb Department of Psychiatry and Biobehavioral Sciences, University of California, Los Angeles, USA.

Kevin J. Mahoney Boston College School of Social, Work Chestnut Hill, USA.

Hoimonty Mazumder Ipas Bangladesh, Dhaka, Bangladesh.

Philip McCallion School of Social Work, College of Public Health, Temple University, Philadelphia, USA.

Jie Mi Department of Intensive Care, The First Affiliated Hospital of Chongqing Medical University, China.

Julie B. Miller AgeLab, Massachusetts Institute of Technology, Cambridge, USA.

Vivian J. Miller Department of Human Services, Bowling Green State University, USA.

Rajean P. Moone College of Continuing and Professional Studies and Center for Healthy Aging and Innovation, University of Minnesota, USA.

Anthony Kwame Morgan Department of Planning, Kwame Nkrumah University of Science and Technology, Kumasi, Ghana.

Nancy Morrow-Howell Brown School and Harvey A. Friedman Center for Aging, Washington University, St. Louis, USA.

Sonia Mukhtar University of Management and Technology, Lahore, Pakistan.

Delores V. Mullings School of Social Work, Memorial University of Newfoundland, St. John's, Canada.

Allison M. Murphy Places for People, Inc., Saint Louis, USA.

Christina Newhill School of Social Work, University of Pittsburgh, Pittsburgh, USA.

Yawen Ning Henry Ford Allegiance Health, Jackson, USA.

Tasmiah Nuzhath Department of Health Promotion and Community Health Sciences, Texas A&M School of Public Health, College Station, USA.

Oluromade Olusa School of Social Work, Social Policy and Social Justice, University College Dublin, Ireland.

Oluwagbemiga Oyinlola Medical Social Services Department, University College Hospital, Ibadan, Nigeria.

Junghyun Park Silver School of Social Work, New York University, New York City, United States.

Taylor R. Patskanick AgeLab, Massachusetts Institute of Technology, Cambridge, USA.

Prince Peprah Social Policy Research Centre, University of New South Wales, Australia.

Tam E. Perry School of Social Work, Wayne State University, Detroit, USA.

Althea Pestine-Stevens School of Social Work, Rutgers, The State University of New Jersey, New Brunswick, USA.

Erica Phillips Cornell Center for Health Equity and Division of General Internal Medicine, Department of Medicine, Weill Cornell Medicine, New York City, USA.

Natalie D. Pope College of Social Work, University of Kentucky College of Social Work, Lexington, USA.

Michelle Putnam School of Social Work, Simmons University, Boston, USA.

Vahid Rashedi School of Behavioral Sciences and Mental Health (Tehran Institute of Psychiatry), Iran University of Medical Sciences, Tehran, Iran.

Mary E. Rauktis School of Social Work, University of Pittsburgh, USA.

Amy R. Roberts Family Studies and Social Work, Miami University, Oxford, Ohio, USA.

Vanessa Rorai Healthier Black Elders Center, Institute of Gerontology, Wayne State University, Detroit, USA.

Claudia Sanford United Community Housing Coalition. Senior Housing Preservation-Detroit, Detroit, USA.

Natsuki Sasaki Places for People, Inc., Saint Louis, USA.

Alexander Seifert University of Applied Sciences and Arts Northwestern Switzerland (FHNW), Olten, Switzerland.

Tracy Schroepfer School of Social Work, University of Wisconsin-Madison, USA.

Penny Shaw Massachusetts Advocates for Nursing Home Reform, Medford, USA.

Huei-Wern Shen Department of Social Work, University of North Texas, USA.

Vineshwar P. Singh School of Medicine, University of Liverpool, England, UK.

Tyler Smathers Wyoming State Hospital, Evanston, USA.

Madeline R. Sterling Cornell Center for Health Equity and Division of General Internal Medicine, Department of Medicine, Weill Cornell Medicine, New York City, USA.

Dan Stewart Human Rights Campaign Foundation, School of Medicine, Boston University Washington D.C., USA.

Madeline Stewart Boston University School of Medicine, Boston, USA.

Abida Sultana Gazi Medical College, Khulna, Bangladesh.

Emma Swinford Harvey A. Friedman Center for Aging, Washington University, St. Louis, USA.

Samia Tasnim Department of Health Promotion and Community Health Sciences, Texas A&M School of Public Health, College Station, USA.

Laura Trejo Los Angeles Community-Academic Partnership for Research in Aging, University of California, USA.

Le Thanh Tung Faculty of Economics and Public Management, Ho Chi Minh City Open University, Ho Chi Minh City, Vietnam.

Soyoon Weon The Korean Ministry of Health and Welfare, Sejong City, South Korea Centre for Research on Children and Families, School of Social Work, McGill University, Montreal, QC, Canada.

Imani Woody Mary's House for Older Adults, Washington, USA.

Xiaoling Xiang University of Michigan School of Social Work, Ann Arbor, USA.

Mingzhao Xiao Department of Urology, The First Affiliated Hospital of Chongqing Medical University, China.

Yan Xie Department of Qinggang Nursing Home, The First Affiliated Hospital of Chongqing Medical University, China.

Mauricio P. Yabar Virginia Commonwealth University School of Social Work, Academic Learning Commons, Richmond, USA.

Xiuli Yu Department of Qinggang Nursing Home, The First Affiliated Hospital of Chongqing Medical University, China.

Olga Yulikova Massachusetts Executive Office of Elder Affairs, Boston, USA.

Qinghua Zhao Department of Nursing, The First Affiliated Hospital of Chongqing Medical University, China.

INTRODUCTION

In December 2019 the novel coronavirus appeared in Wuhan, China and COVID-19 became the named disease associated with this virus in January 2020. The rapid spread of the novel coronavirus (SARS-CoV-2) has resulted in the global pandemic of COVID-19 with more than 34 million cases worldwide and over 1,009,000 deaths from the disease (Johns Hopkins University, 2020) at the time of this writing. Infection and mortality rates differ across nations. Data on the virus spread, as well as death attribution, is believed to be significantly under counted and reported (WHO, 2020a), by perhaps a factor of ten in the United States (Havers et al., 2020), one of the nations with the worst viral outbreak.

Sudharsanan et al. (2020) conducted a multi-national analysis of age-adjusted case fatality across 95 nations that considered their varying age-specific population distributions. They found that population age distribution accounts for 66% of the variance in national case fatality rates – with nations with a greater proportion of older adults having higher fatality rates. Although they and others (Angelopoulos et al., 2020) caution that testing bias toward older adults and persons with more severe symptoms exits in many nations (and individuals with mild or moderate symptoms go untested) and may inflate the proportion of different age groups who are counted as COVID-19 positive -thus influencing incidence and mortality rates. That said, there remains clear evidence that older adults who contract COVID-19 are much more likely to die from the disease than middle-aged, younger adults or children (CDC, 2020; Klug, 2020a). Older adults remain statistically more likely to develop severe COVID-19 symptoms and to be hospitalized at disproportionate rates compared to other age groups (Shahid et al., 2020). About 75% of COVID-19 fatalities in the United States are adults age 65 and older (Wortham et al., 2020) and this pattern exists worldwide with estimates as high as 90% of all COVID-19 deaths occurring within the older adult population (Klug, 2020a). Additionally, global evidence is building that health disparities and structural inequalities resulting from racism and prejudice have contributed to worse outcomes among non-majority populations and/or populations sub-groups in the United States and United Kingdom (Bhala et al., 2020), Brazil (Baqui et al., 2020) and other nations (Lloyd-Sherlock et al., 2020). This includes worse outcomes among older adults in sub-groups who have experience life-long inequalities and marginalization and also experience ageism.

Ageism existed prior to emergence of SARS-CoV-2 but has been more widely exposed during this pandemic. This is perhaps seen most blatantly in guidelines that suggest rationing or limiting care for older adults and persons with disabilities, such as those initially forwarded in Italy at the beginning of their viral outbreak (Cesari & Proietti, 2020). But also evident in the wildfire-like spread of COVID-19 in nursing homes and older adult care homes world-wide which has brought a stronger spotlight to long-standing concerns about self-determination, choice of care location, availability and affordability of care services, and quality of care for older adults with functional limitations and social care needs (Klug, 2020b). In the ongoing analysis of the impact of the COVID-19 pandemic, the intersections of ageism, health disparities and structural inequalities should and will be investigated and considered. However, the roots of each of these phenomena run deep and what will be focused on in a sustained way during the current phase of the pandemic and post-pandemic remains to be seen.

The *Journal of Gerontological Social Work (JGSW)* put out a call for letters to the editor and commentaries in the beginning of the pandemic with the aim of providing a venue for scholars, particularly social work scholars, to highlight issues and concerns related to social work practice with older adults, the care and treatment of older adults, and social, economic and environmental factors affecting older adults as they experience this early era of the novel coronavirus and COVID-19. We received submissions from around the world and have pulled them together into this special collection. We recognize that not all issues, concerns or voices are represented here. The incredible disruption COVD-19 has created in individual lives and in communities has not spared scholars, researchers, or educators. In particular we acknowledge that individuals with fewer health, social and economic resources; individuals who are members of marginalized population groups or those experiencing discrimination; individuals with work, family, professional, and community responsibilities that require attention and care; and individuals with other obligations and needs may have desired to, but not have been able to, contribute to these calls. We remain open to hearing their voices and always encourage the submission of thoughtful manuscripts related to the pandemic including commentaries, research articles, policy analyses, media reviews, and other types of work to *JGSW*.

This special collection opens with a series of commentaries that focus on gerontological social work's response to COVID-19. These are followed by letters to the editor which have been placed into several sections: Gerontological social work role in addressing COVID-19, COVID-19 and social work with diverse groups, COVID-19 and health and social care, Social isolation and the digital experience in COVID-19, and Interventions to support older adults during COVID-19.

Commentary and letter authors were unified in their emphasis on the important role social workers have played and/or can play in directly supporting older adults, addressing community-level service and support needs of older adults and their families, and advocating for and facilitating policy solutions that value older adults and care providers. Themes that emerged across letters include:

- The importance of advancing gerontological social work education and training as so few professionals are specifically trained to work with older adults, yet the disease effects on older adults have been the greatest.
- The need to actively address ageism and disease-related stigma as the value of life based on age, disability, and disease status has been openly discussed by decision makers and professionals during the pandemic in ways that suggest the value of older adults is less than other age groups.
- The requirement of social workers to call attention to social and economic injustices – including discriminatory practices and poor treatment of marginalized populations – and actively work to support these groups through the pandemic as well as to address the individual, community, and structural factors that create excess and unnecessary vulnerability to disease.
- The need to advance home and community-based long-term care or social care as a means of increasing an individual's choice, control, and self-determination and reducing the risk of older adults to COVID-19 and other known negative institutional outcomes.
- Concern about the effects on older adults of social isolation, loneliness and exclusion that have come with social distancing practices and the further movement to an all digital and remote-engagement world and the importance of remedying these.
- The importance of drawing on and amplifying awareness of existing knowledge and known solutions as well as innovating when needed to meet the needs of older adults and their families as we move through this pandemic.
- The globally shared concerns about the health and wellness of older adults and the important role gerontological social workers have worldwide in supporting older adults and their families at the micro, mezzo and macro levels.

Together, these themes help to set the direction for future gerontological social work related to the COVID-19 pandemic and beyond. As noted previously, the voices in this issue only represent a small portion of those in the field, but the messages they put forth reflect the values that are core to gerontological social work practice. The commentaries and letters in this special collection capture this unprecedented moment in time when the SARS-CoV-2 virus connects us all in profound ways and demonstrate the important role gerontological social workers have in helping to solve problems, large and small, that the pandemic has created and exacerbated.

We thank all of the authors who responded to *JGSW*'s special call and shared their thoughts with us and our readers. It has been our privilege to compile your voices into this issue.

We wish you good health,

Michelle Putnam

Huei-Wern Shen

References

Angelopoulos, A. N., Pathak, R., Varma, R., & Jordan, M. I. (2020). On identifying and mitigating bias in the estimation of the COVID-19 case fatality rate. *Harvard Data Science Review*. https://doi.org/10.1162/99608f92.f01ee285

Baqui, P., Bica, I., Marra, V., Ercole, A., & van der Schaar, M. (2020). Ethnic and regional variations in hospital mortality from COVID-19 in Brazil: A cross-sectional observational study. *The Lancet. Global Health*, 8(8), e1018–e1026. https://doi.org/10.1016/S2214-109X(20)30285-0

Bhala, N., Curry, G., Martineau, A. R., Agyemang, C., & Bhopal, R. (2020). Sharpening the global focus on ethnicity and race in the time of COVID-19. *Lancet (London, England)*, 395 (10238), 1673–1676. https://doi.org/10.1016/S0140-6736(20)31102-8

CDC. (2020). *Weekly updates by select demographic and geographic characteristics provisional death counts for coronavirus disease 2019 (COVID-19)*. https://www.cdc.gov/nchs/nvss/vsrr/covid_weekly/index.htm

Cesari, M., & Proietti, M. (2020). COVID-19 in Italy: Ageism and decision making in a pandemic. *Journal of the American Medical Directors Association*, 21(5), 576–577. https://doi.org/10.1016/j.jamda.2020.03.025

Havers, F. P., Reed, C., Lim, T., Montgomery, J. M., Klena, J. D., Hall, A. J., Fry, A. M., Cannon, D. L., Chiang, C. F., Gibbons, A., Krapiunaya, I., Morales-Betoulle, M., Roguski, K., Rasheed, M., Freeman, B., Lester, S., Mills, L., Carroll, D. S., Owen, S. M., Johnson, J. A., & Thornburg, N. J. (2020). Seroprevalence of antibodies to SARS-CoV-2 in 10 sites in the United States, March 23-May 12, 2020. *JAMA Internal Medicine*. https://doi.org/10.1001/jamainternmed.2020.4130

Johns Hopkins University. (2020, July 29). *Coronavirus Resource Center, COVID-19 Dashboard*. https://coronavirus.jhu.edu/map.html

Klug, H. H. (2020a, April 2). *Statement – Older people are at highest risk from COVID-19, but all must act to prevent community spread*. WHO (World Health Organization). https://www.euro.who.int/en/health-topics/health-emergencies/coronavirus-covid-19/statements/statement-older-people-are-at-highest-risk-from-covid-19,-but-all-must-act-to-prevent-community-spread

Klug, H. H. (2020b, April 2). *Statement – Invest in the overlooked and unsung: Build sustainable people-centred long-term care in the wake of COVID-19*. WHO (World Health Organization). https://www.euro.who.int/en/media-centre/sections/statements/2020/statement-invest-in-the-overlooked-and-unsung-build-sustainable-people-centred-long-term-care-in-the-wake-of-covid–19

Lloyd-Sherlock, P., Ebrahim, S., Geffen, L., & McKee, M. (2020). Bearing the brunt of covid-19: Older people in low and middle income countries. *BMJ (Clinical Research Ed.)*, *368*, m1052. https://doi.org/10.1136/bmj.m1052

Shahid, Z., Kalayanamitra, R., McClafferty, B., Kepko, D., Ramgobin, D., Patel, R., Aggarwal, C. S., Vunnam, R., Sahu, N., Bhatt, D., Jones, K., Golamari, R., & Jain, R. (2020). COVID-19 and older adults: What we know. *Journal of the American Geriatrics Society*, *68*(5), 926–929. https://doi.org/10.1111/jgs.16472

Sudharsanan, N., Didzun, O., Bärnighausen, T., & Geldsetzer, P. (2020). The contribution of the age distribution of cases to COVID-19 case fatality across countries: A 9-country demographic study. *Annals of Internal Medicine*, 10.7326/M20-2973. Advance online publication. https://doi.org/10.7326/M20-2973

WHO (World Health Organization). (2020a). *Coronavirus disease (COVID-19) situation report – 190*. https://www.who.int/docs/default-source/coronaviruse/situation-reports/20200728-covid-19-sitrep-190.pdf?sfvrsn=fec17314_2

Wortham, J. M., Lee, J. T., Althomsons, S., Latash, J., Davidson, A., Guerra, K., Murray, K., McGibbon, E., Pichardo, C., Toro, B., Li, L., Paladini, M., Eddy, M. L., Reilly, K. H., McHugh, L., Thomas, D., Tsai, S., Ojo, M., Rolland, S., Bhat, M., & Reagan-Steiner, S. (2020). Characteristics of persons who died with COVID-19 - United States, February 12-May 18, 2020. *MMWR. Morbidity and Mortality Weekly Report*, *69*(28), 923–929. https://doi.org/10.15585/mmwr.mm6928e1

Part I

Commentaries on Gerontological Social Work's Response to COVID-19

The Consequences of Ageist Language are upon us

Clara Berridge (iD) and Nancy Hooyman

ABSTRACT

The COVID–19 pandemic has highlighted the ease in which ageist language is employed and ageist stereotypes are used to characterize older adults. These are harmful and display an impressive lack of future thinking – as younger and middle-aged adults who use this language and forward these concepts also hope to live long lives. The disproportionately negative outcomes for older adults in this pandemic in part, reflect social and economic inequalities that are manifest throughout the life course of marginalized groups including persons of color. They also reflect major problems with institutional living be it in prisons or nursing homes. Social workers and allied professionals can work to address these manifestations of ageism in part by employing inclusive language – as advised by the Reframing Aging Project, working to build and support strong intergenerational relationships, working to eradicate social and economic disparities at all life stages, and advocating for a more critical look at institutionalization of older adults.

"if you guys know any uh, uh, the elderly, any older people that may need help, please call them, check on them, see if they need anything … Not an old, help an old person, uh, yeah, help an elderly uh person, yeah, ok."

-Jimmy Fallon, The Tonight Show: Home Edition, March 19 (00:35–00:58)

When Jimmy Fallon stumbled over his description of the population experiencing higher mortality rates from COVID-19, it was a telling moment. One of us is a baby boomer and the other a millennial-Gen X cusper. As gerontologists in the city where the virus first touched down in the U.S., we were concerned by the widespread use of "the elderly" in the media because it undermines cross-generational solidarity.

Referring to *the* elderly as a homogenous mass is ageism, attributing characteristics to all members of a group because of the shared trait of age. We offer three distinct reasons for not using "the elderly" in the context of the pandemic:

(1) It turns people off, stokes generational conflict, and is not specific, causing confusion in public health messaging.
(2) It masks racial disparities in access to health care and underlying health conditions that impact outcomes of COVID-19.
(3) This ageist language plays into age- and disability-based triage policies in hospitals.

We address counterproductive language and draw on the research-based national Reframing Aging Initiative to suggest how best to talk about these issues, while acknowledging the potential hollowness that "we are all in this together" in the face of disparate impacts of the pandemic as well as the need for structural changes to benefit the essential direct care workforce.

After our Governor Jay Inslee issued recommendations for people 60+ to be the only groups to isolate at home, media reports rarely identified this specific age category, but instead only referenced "seniors" or *the* "elderly." Five years ago, the editor of this journal announced the replacement of "the elderly" with "older adults" and required qualification when "vulnerable" is used. The *Journal of Gerontological Social Work* was ahead of others in avoiding these vague and problematic descriptors (Putnam, 2015). Now, the American Geriatrics Society requires authors to use precise age ranges (Lundebjerg, Trucil, Hammond, & Applegate, 2017).

During a public health crisis, such clarity is particularly urgent. A 62- or 67-year-old who reads "senior" or "the elderly" may not think the guidelines apply to them. But that's not really an issue of denial or internalized ageism on their part. The older adult population refers generally to people 65+, covering more than one generation and age cohort, so it makes sense that we'd confront language issues when attempting to describe this very large and diverse population. The population age 65–115 is more heterogeneous than any other age group (Lowsky, Olshansky, Bhattacharya, & Goldman, 2014), from marathon runners to people living with severe emphysema, so it is not surprising that people resist direction based on an arbitrary chronological marker. "The elderly" is what our colleague Wendy Lustbader calls an empty category. That is, people don't identify with this word. "The elderly" is associated with frailty and accompanying paternalism. Berridge recently pointed out in *The Atlantic* that "The fact that people don't often voluntarily relate to this term is a strong reason to not apply it to them" (Pinsker, 2020).

As disability justice activist Lydia X.Z. Brown notes in their blog on ableist language, discussions of language should include critique of the larger system of oppression (Brown, 2014). Ageism is discrimination against older people due to negative and inaccurate stereotypes. It can limit a person's opportunities for meaningful employment (Kita, 2019) and other forms of productivity and negatively affect health (Adler, 2013). It also masks dramatic racial inequities among older adults that lead to a disparate incidence of heart and lung diseases – risk factors for serious illness and mortality from COVID-19 (Jordan & Oppel, 2020).

There is an abundance of evidence that race and experiences of discrimination negatively impact health outcomes, and the ways in which COVID-19 differentially harms Black, Latinx, and Native people are painfully visible. In a recent discussion for *Social Work Today*, V. Nikki Jones outlines reasons why the pandemic is hitting African Americans in the U.S. especially hard, including barriers to the social determinants of good health (economic stability, education, social and community context, health and health care, and neighborhood and built environment). She explains that these are linked to cultural memory and historical trauma. Another key factor is African Americans' role in what is now referred to as the essential workforce, built on a history of economic exploitation (Jones, 2020). In a Working Paper published by the Harvard Center for Population and Development Studies in April, Jarvis Chen and Nancy Krieger report findings from county level data that "people living in the most impoverished, crowded, and racially and economically polarized counties are experiencing substantially elevated rates of COVID-19 infection and death," including a 6-fold greater rate of death for populations living in counties where 61–100% of the population is of color than those living in counties where less than 17.3% of the population is of color (Chen & Krieger, 2020).

As with other forms of oppression, ageism has a tendency to naturalize inequities. Vulnerability becomes biological and acceptable. It's important to ask in what ways vulnerability is socially constructed. At the time of publishing, one-third of coronavirus deaths in this country have occurred among nursing home residents and workers (Yourish, Lai, Ivory, & Smith, 2020). While older adults as a whole are more vulnerable to negative outcomes from the virus, either because of age-associated changes to their immune systems or because of underlying conditions (The American Federation for Aging Research, 2020), those who are living in these facilities are made far more vulnerable by the arrangement of aggregate care provided in close quarters – often without private rooms and in understaffed conditions. Further, there has been loud outcry by prison abolitionists and reformers about unsanitary and cramped conditions faced by people incarcerated in prisons and jails and thus more vulnerable to the virus (Li & Lewis, 2020). Incarcerated individuals, including those over age 55, are disproportionately Black and Latinx people who are likely to have faced years of health care disparities, compounding their risk for contracting and experiencing negative effects of COVID-19.

Comorbidities are often consequences of social determinants of health. As such, hospital triage during the pandemic is problematic when it is based on comorbidities that influence expected survival. Others have described how ageism pairs with ableism to potentially deprioritize people in line to receive life-saving care (Kukla, 2020; Ayalon, Chasteen, Diehl, et al., 2020). In a recent panel on disability and COVID-19 (Student Disability Commission, 2020), philosophy scholar Joe Stramondo points out that the disability paradox – in which nondisabled people would rate one's quality of life lower than disabled people do – isn't a paradox at all, but rather, a consequence of disability stigma. And these ideas about quality of life get translated into triage policies. Stramondo also observes, as disability justice activists have, that our capitalist economy's emphasis on productivity underlies beliefs about the value of peoples' lives. Stramondo explains, "In practice our elders and disabled people are warehoused in nursing homes and other institutions. In more theoretical terms this kind of thing happens because of beliefs about people not being productive enough within a capitalist society." In gerontology, we see this appeal to productivity and independence reflected in the productive and successful aging discourses (Berridge & Martison, 2018; Martinson & Berridge, 2015).

The intergenerational tensions stoked by this pandemic have intensified, with millennials and baby boomers sparring over who was crowding Florida beaches and who doesn't need to be instructed by their children to stay home (Schulman, 2020). Having others repeatedly tell them what to do angers some older adults and makes some feel stigmatized. The fear underlying adult children's concern for parents – who they are not yet prepared to lose – is also legitimate. Millennials would benefit from understanding how ageism is at play when they interfere with their parents' autonomous decision making. That feeling of disrespect and paternalism can be painfully familiar and touches a nerve because it reeks of ageism. Cross-generational learning teaches us not to be shortsighted: In the next pandemic, millennials may find themselves in the vulnerable category (Yong, 2020).

Othering language like "the elderly" positions older people as a separate social group apart from "the rest of us." But this conflicts with our interdependent lives and cross-generational care experiences. Twenty percent of U.S. households are multigenerational (Fry, 2019), and 3 million older adults are raising grandchildren (Allen, 2018; Pittman, 2015). The language of ageism also interferes with collective action for core principles (nondiscrimination, equality) and the greater good (Eligon & Burch, 2020; Ne'eman, 2020). It doesn't help when geriatricians and other experts in the health sciences use "the elderly" in media interviews. Jane Aronson's NY Times op-ed draws attention to overlooked ageist policies (Trump's deregulation of the nursing home industry) and the pervasive ageism underlying cruel "boomer remover" memes, but she inadvertently invokes othering when using "the elderly" in the same piece (Aronson,

2020). If the media and expert interviewees used a stronger message of collectivity, generational tensions might be eased. Older adults are more likely to act upon the public health imperative of self-quarantine when presented in terms of risks faced by adults of all ages who have compromised immune systems or underlying lung or heart conditions, not just those of a certain age (Kukla, 2020).

The consequences of ageist language are upon us, but we can address counterproductive language choices. The Gerontological Society of America promotes the Reframing Aging Project recommendations to use older people instead of "senior" and "the elderly" and use inclusive "we" and "us" terms (FrameWorks Institute). This dynamic project is posting language suggestions every few days for reporting on COVID-19 to help everyone "amplify the values of justice, inclusion, and interdependence" (FrameWorks Institute, 2020b). Antidotes to us-vs-them thinking include writing about how we are all in this together and our need to hold our representatives accountable to democratic ideals (Bruni, 2020). On the other hand, statements of togetherness can start to seem superficial when inequities by race and disability are minimized or overlooked.

And not to pick on Jimmy Fallon. It's not all his fault that he couldn't spit it out. The following day he featured singer J Balvin, who gave a shout out to The National Domestic Workers Alliance, a cross-generational solidarity organization that uplifts skilled care work performed by home care aides and nurses' aides. Our ties of interdependence can no longer be overlooked as we are all depending on both the young and old who comprise this critical workforce that is typically underpaid and undervalued (Jamison, 2020). While the media and public are giving greater recognition and thanks to this hands-on workforce, what will matter over time is whether structural changes are made to ensure a living wage and safe work conditions.

References

Adler, T. (2013). Ageism: Alive and Kicking. Association for Psychological Science. https://www.psycho logicalscience.org/observer/ageism-alive-and-kicking

Allen, K. (2018). Grandparents Report Success in Raising Grandchildren. AARP: https://www.aarp.org/ home-family/friends-family/info-2018/grandparents-raising-kids.html

Aronson, L. (2020). 'Covid-19 Kills Only Old People.' Only?. The New York Times. https://www. nytimes.com/2020/03/22/opinion/coronavirus-elderly.html?smid=tw-share&fbclid= IwAR1chQPRrNoi4dGXZ2ju73-6ddvgUu8i4n5dVMik08BuQlaDFSJa3IoUz2o

Ayalon, L, Chasteen, A, Diehl, M, Levy, B, Neupert, S. D, Rothermund, K, Tesch-Römer, C, & Wahl, H. (2020). Aging in times of the covid-19 pandemic: avoiding ageism and fostering intergenerational solidarity. *The Journals Of Gerontology: Series B*. doi:10.1093/geronb/gbaa051

Berridge, C, & Martinson, Marty. (2018). Valuing old age without leveraging ableism. *Generations, 41*(4), 83-91.

Brown, L. X. Z. (2014). Violence in Language: Circling Back to Linguistic Ableism. Autistic Hoya Blog. https://www.autistichoya.com/2014/02/violence-linguistic-ableism.html

Bruni, F. (2020). We're relying on trump to care about our lives. The New York Times. https://www. nytimes.com/2020/03/24/opinion/coronavirus-trump-economy.html

Chen, J. T., & Krieger, K. (2020). Revealing the unequal burden of COVID-19 by income, race/ ethnicity, and household crowding: US county vs. ZIP code analyses. Harvard Center for Population and Development Studies Working Paper, 19 (1). https://cdn1.sph.harvard.edu/wp-content/uploads/sites/ 1266/2020/04/HCPDS_Volume-19_No_1_20_covid19_RevealingUnequalBurden_ HCPDSWorkingPaper_04212020-1.pdf

Eligon, J., & Burch, A. D. S. (2020). Questions of bias in covid-19 treatment add to the mourning for black families. The New York Times. https://www.nytimes.com/2020/05/10/us/coronavirus-african-americans-bias.html

FrameWorks Institute. (2020a). Reframing aging. https://frameworksinstitute.org/reframing-aging.html

FrameWorks Institute. (2020b). Framing covid-19. http://frameworksinstitute.org/framing-covid-19. html

Fry, R. (2019). The number of people in the average U.S. household is going up for the first time in over 160 years. Pew Research Center. https://www.pewresearch.org/fact-tank/2019/10/01/the-number-of-people-in-the-average-u-s-household-is-going-up-for-the-first-time-in-over-160-years/

Jamison, P. (2020). Unprotected and unprepared: Home health aides who care for sick, elderly brace for covid-19. The Washington Post. https://www-washingtonpost-com.cdn.ampproject.org/c/s/www.washingtonpost.com/dc-md-va/2020/03/23/home-health-care-aides-coronavirus-elderly/?outputType=amp&fbclid=IwAR3kd-Fgh4DbH3OaG6ATBprEdpudlcEBr4XUbcHE6YU6UQAxt-Ei2Fq9gzU

Jones, V. N. (2020). Why african americans are hardest hit by covid-19. Social Work Today. https://www.socialworktoday.com/archive/exc_042120.shtml?fbclid=IwAR08DIJCKS_W8ibsiEbTM0Uls0ZbbWu_M9nGkywKdPg5CdTq2ik6r2GVEPI

Jordan, M., & Oppel, R. A., Jr. (2020). For Latinos and COVID-19, Doctors are Seeing an 'Alarming' Disparity. The New York Times. https://www.nytimes.com/2020/05/07/us/coronavirus-latinos-disparity.html

Kita, J. (2019). Workplace age discrimination still flourishes in america. AARP. https://www.aarp.org/work/working-at-50-plus/info-2019/age-discrimination-in-america.html

Kukla, E. (2020). My life is more 'disposable' during this pandemic. The New York Times. https://www.nytimes.com/2020/03/19/opinion/coronavirus-disabled-health-care.html

Lai, Yourish, K., Ivory, R.K.K., & Smith, D., M. (2020). One-Third of All U.S. Coronavirus Deaths Are Nursing Home Residents or Workers. The New York Times. https://www.nytimes.com/interactive/2020/05/09/us/coronavirus-cases-nursing-homes-us.html?fbclid=IwAR3-zYgnmvF6wut9-Jd_-FiMyWiIBV403ES8TEU5FNfXD2519jGwfDmAEZc

Li, W., & Lewis, N. (2020). This chart shows why the prison population is so vulnerable to covid-19. The Marshall Project. https://www.themarshallproject.org/2020/03/19/this-chart-shows-why-the-prison-population-is-so-vulnerable-to-covid-19

Lowsky, D. J, Olshansky, S. J, Bhattacharya, J, & Goldman, D. P. (2014). Heterogeneity in healthy aging. the journals of gerontology. *The Journals Of Gerontology Series A: Biological Sciences and Medical Sciences, 69*(6), 640–649. doi: 10.1093/gerona/glt162

Lundebjerg, N.E, Trucil, D.E, Hammond, E.C, & Applegate, W.B. (2017). when it comes to older adults, language matters: journal of the american geriatrics society adopts modified american medical association style. *Journal Of The American Geriatrics Society Adopts Modified American Medical Association Style, 65* (7), 1386-1388. doi: 10.1111/jgs.2017.65.issue-7

Martinson, M, & Berridge, C. (2015). Successful aging and its discontents: a systematic review of the social gerontology literature. *The Gerontologist, 55*(1), 58-69. doi:10.1093/geront/gnu037

Ne'eman, A. (2020). 'I Will Not Apologize for My Needs.' The New York Times. https://www.nytimes.com/2020/03/23/opinion/coronavirus-ventilators-triage-disability.html?fbclid=IwAR2roieISQuDL8U7AKxe3VSZ0psVGSUJaFf3ICJOnWKkAuEaspdWf_POKmE

Pinsker, J. (2020). When does someone become 'old'? the atlantic. https://www.theatlantic.com/family/archive/2020/01/old-people-older-elderly-middle-age/605590/

Pittman, L. (2015). How well does the "safety net" work for family safety nets? economic survival strategies among grandmother caregivers in severe deprivation. *Rsf: The Russell Sage Foundation Journal Of The Social Sciences, 1*(1), 78–97. doi:10.7758/rsf.2015.1.1.05

Putnam, M. (2015). Replacing the elderly with older adults in jgsw publications. *Journal Of Gerontological Social Work, 58*(3), 229-231. doi: 10.1080/01634372.2015.1033363

Schulman, M. (2020). Convincing boomer parents to take the coronavirus seriously. The New Yorker. https://www.newyorker.com/culture/culture-desk/convincing-boomer-parents-to-take-the-coronavirus-seriously

Student Disability Commission (University of Washington). (2020). Ableism and coronavirus webinar. Recording retrieved. http://sdc.asuw.org/events/ableism-and-coronavirus-webinar/

The American Federation for Aging Research (AFAR) (April 15), (2020). Why aging immune systems are more vulnerable to the coronavirus. Next Avenue. https://www.nextavenue.org/immune-systems-vulnerable-coronavirus/?fbclid=IwAR2MHba9W0wz8AuifQS74YREem90nrV1D_H62TFeXeznImMKLwcG2UFlS94

Yong, E. (2020). How the pandemic will end. The Atlantic. https://www.theatlantic.com/health/archive/2020/03/how-will-coronavirus-end/608719/

Applying Gerontological Social Work Perspectives to the Coronavirus Pandemic

Emma Swinford, Natalie Galucia, and Nancy Morrow-Howell

ABSTRACT

Social workers are familiar with the challenges brought on by the coronavirus pandemic; and we apply three gerontological social work perspectives that might increase our chances of minimizing negative outcomes and improving health and quality of life for everyone. First, the reality that the older population is very heterogeneous challenges ageism and age-stereotyping that has surfaced with COVID-19. Second, concepts of cumulative disadvantage and intersectionality offer clear explanations of the disparities that are being illuminated and lead us to advocate for fundamental changes to reduce disparities in later life and for people across the life course. Third, a strength-based perspective highlights the assets of the older population and the opportunities for positive developments coming out of the crisis. We can capitalize on momentum to increase advance care planning, to reduce social isolation, and expand the use of on-line technology for service provision. We can bolster our arguments to support older workers, volunteers, and caregivers. The fact that these social work perspectives are so applicable to the coronavirus situation reminds us of their fundamental relevance. Gerontological social work has much to offer in our roles as researchers, educators, practitioners, and advocates during this crisis, and our foundational principles serve us well.

Introduction

Some of the challenges our country is facing because of the coronavirus pandemic are new, but many are familiar to social workers. Social workers practice across all of the arenas that people currently struggle with as a result of COVID-19: health and mental health, unemployment, and economic insecurity, family stress, caregiving arrangements, and more. Social workers bring a commitment to social justice and health equity throughout these practices. Thus, social workers, and in particular, gerontological social workers, bring valuable perspectives to efforts to adjust to and recover from the pandemic. If we apply three foundational gerontological social work perspectives to the current situation, we might improve our chances of minimizing negative outcomes and improving health and quality of life for everyone. These three guiding ideas are: (1) the older population is very heterogeneous; (2) a life time of disadvantages cumulate to threaten the well-being of all people in later life, especially older adults of color and lower socioeconomic status; and (3) a strength-based perspective enables us to see opportunities for growth and positive development. This commentary highlights these three social work perspectives and how they relate to our current situation.

Heterogeneity of the older adult population

Negative sentiments toward the older population began alongside the first reports of the coronavirus. The World Health Organization's Director-General admonished governments that were slow to react to the virus, accusing them of downplaying the threat because it was anticipated to largely affect older populations (Barnes, 2020). There were alarming reports from Alabama of age-discriminatory ventilator policies (Ault, 2020). Dan Patrick, the Lieutenant Governor of Texas, indicated that older people should consider sacrificing themselves for the economy (Sonmez, 2020). #Boomremover appeared in the social media.

These ageist ideas are based on damaging age stereotypes which reduce an extremely heterogenous group into a single cohort. The COVID-19 pandemic has led the public to view the older population as one monolithic group, seen as vulnerable, in need of special concern, and concentrated in nursing homes. The reality, however, is that older adults have an extremely diverse set of characteristics, backgrounds, capabilities, and desires. It is a dynamic population that includes people in a 40+ year age range. The field of social work honors the heterogeneity of this group by emphasizing the importance of individual experience rather than categorizations (National Association of Social Workers Delegate Assembly, 2017).

It is true that age is positively associated with infection, severity of illness, and mortality in this pandemic – older people are more susceptible to poor outcomes. These trends are based more specifically on underlying chronic illnesses and weaker immune systems, two conditions that are associated with, but not equal to, age. The public widely assumes that as chronological age goes up, health inevitably declines, but nearly three-quarters of adults over 65 reported no health-based limitations with their work or housework (Lowsky, 2014). Thus, we need to recognize that vulnerability to viral infection varies across the older population, and younger adults are at risk as well. In fact, as gerontologists, it is interesting to hear stories of centenarians who lived through the Spanish flu epidemic in 1918 and recently survived being infected with the coronavirus (Miller, 2020).

A further testimony to the heterogeneity of the older population is the reality that older people engage in variety of critical roles during this pandemic. Older adults are part of the frontline workforce dealing with this crisis by virtue of the fact that nearly a quarter of the U.S. workforce is over the age of 55 (U.S. Bureau of Labor Statistics, n.d.). Older adults work in all sectors of our economy; and actually, older adults drive the economy through consumer spending; 56 cents of every dollar is spent by someone over the age of 50 (Accius & Suh, 2019). Joe Coughlin (Coughlin & Yoquinto, 2020) aptly observes "You can't choose the economy over Grandma, it turns out, because, in a very real sense, Grandma *is* the economy – and that's doubly true in rural regions and retirement destinations."

It is well documented that older adults contribute substantial hours of their time to nonprofit and public organizations meeting community needs ("Health Benefits of Senior Corps," 2018). The pandemic has brought shelter-in-place guidelines and closures of many service organizations; and many older adults have been unable to perform their normal volunteer duties. This is not only a loss to the community, but also to older adults' sense of purpose and contribution, though many are continuing to find ways to donate their time. AARP released a Community Connections tool to help older adults find volunteer opportunities near them and set up mutual aid funds for their communities (Markowitz, 2020). Older people are leading efforts to tutor children remotely, to make masks, to raise money for food banks, and to provide telephone reassurance to isolated people (Liska, 2020; The Eisner Foundation, 2020). It is advised that all of us, regardless of age, begin planning how we will resume and increase our service efforts when we can return to these vital roles.

Although volunteer roles have been disrupted, family caregiving and helping friends and neighbors continue. As we know, many older Americans provide unpaid caregiving services to family members and friends; over one-third of care-givers in the United States are over the age of 65 (Family Caregiver Alliance, 2019). The disruptions to usual care have made the provision of supportive assistance in personal care, meal preparation, and medication management particularly difficult. For some, routine grandparenting roles have been altered due to social distancing guidelines; but for many grandparents, childcare continues and is more demanding with home-schooling responsibilities and continual family proximity.

In sum, as gerontological social workers, we know that chronological age is a widely used, poor indicator of a person's health and functioning. We must emphasize that age-based criteria for dealing with the virus and assessing contribution to the common good in this time of crisis are dangerous. We must continually remind people that there is great heterogeneity in the older population and spotlight the contributions of older people as workers, volunteers, community members, and care-givers. We should not let sweeping generalizations of aging obscure the tangible and intangible impacts that older adults have on our society.

Cumulative disadvantage and intersectionality

The coronavirus pandemic is exposing deep-seated racial and socioeconomic disparities in our society – disparities that have always been the concern of the social work profession. Gerontological social workers in particular understand how injustices and inequalities follow a person into later life and play out in old age. Our concepts about cumulative disadvantage and intersectionality describe the current situation accurately, as certain groups of older adults entered the pandemic with an already increased risk of negative outcomes. People who have experienced discrimination and marginalization in education, employment, housing, and health care across the life course are at high risk for poor health and economic outcomes at older ages; and racial, ethnic, gender, and socioeconomic status overlap to exacerbate the struggle to live safe and healthy lives in later years. We are seeing these forces play out on a daily basis during this pandemic.

Nationally, Black Americans comprise 13% of the U.S. population, but represent 33% of COVID-19 hospitalizations (Maqbool, 2020). For example, just 14% of Michigan's population is African-American, but this population makes up 33% of infections and 40% of deaths (Taylor, 2020). The disproportionate burden of negative health outcomes from COVID-19 in communities of color has multiple roots. Health care facilities and testing centers are less accessible in predominantly minority neighborhoods (Reid, 2020; Taylor, 2020). African-Americans are less likely to have health insurance than white Americans, creating a barrier to routine and emergency care (Sohn, 2017). Studies have shown that the implicit biases of healthcare professionals negatively impact the type and quality of care that African-American patients receive (Taylor, 2020). Older African-Americans are at higher risk of diabetes and heart disease, underlying conditions that lead to poor survival from COVID-19 (Carnethon et al., 2017; Hargrave, 2010).

Low-income populations and communities of color are being hit hardest by the coronavirus due to disparities in employment. Recent data indicate that 14% more black workers had been laid off or had hours cut than white workers (Kurtzleben, 2020). Less than 20% of African-Americans are able to stay home and keep their jobs (Taylor, 2020). Low-wage workers are less likely to have paid sick time, so many must continue to work, despite exposure risk (Morath & Feintzeig, 2020). As we have seen by infection rates of residents and staff in nursing homes, paid caregivers in the long-term care industry are choosing between an income or protecting themselves by staying home (Chen, 2020). We have yet to see all of these data presented by age cross-tabulated with race and sex, and these analyses are needed to clearly elucidate the mounting disparities. However, we know that older people are among these low-wage workers and unpaid caregivers, and they carry the disproportionate burden of having more chronic health conditions that increase the risk for negative outcomes.

Throughout history, the disproportionate burdens brought on by natural disasters have revealed how racism and classism intersect to place people at risk in later life. We saw this during the Chicago heat wave, when poor and isolated older people accounted for the majority of deaths (Klinenberg, 2002); and again with Hurricane Katrina, where almost 50% of deaths were among people 75 years and older, and where residents of nursing homes were left uncared for (Brunkard et al., 2008; Dosa et al., 2010). The coronavirus pandemic has placed society at a similar juncture again. We have clear evidence of the cumulative disadvantage and intersectionality that we are familiar with as gerontologists; we hope that this time, the general public and public officials will pay attention, understand this reality more clearly, and take action. As gerontological social workers, we know that system changes in education, employment, and health care are needed for children and adults to ensure quality of life for all of us when we are old. We have a unique moment in time to educate and advocate for fundamental changes to reduce disparities in later life and for people across the life course, and we should not let it slip away.

Strength-based perspective

The field of social work is driven by a strengths-based perspective and social workers are trained to look for assets and opportunities, even in the most challenging of circumstances. Applying this lens to the current pandemic allows us to build on what we are seeing to increase visibility of important issues, advocate for resources, and take advantage of momentum to advance positive change. We outline several of these opportunities below.

Advance care planning

For years, health care professionals and advocates have encouraged people to consider and share their preferences for end-of-life care and decision-making. A 2017 report states that while just over half of Americans have had conversations about their wishes for end-of-life medical care with a loved one, only 11% have discussed their preferences with a health care professional. Among those who had spoken with a loved one, only 27% have their desires documented in writing. The most commonly cited reason for having not done formal advance care planning (72%) was simply not having gotten around to it (Hamel, 2017).

The coronavirus pandemic has inserted a degree of urgency and necessity into end-of-life care conversations and consequently, there has been a surge of interest in advance care planning. The Conversation Project partnered with Ariadne Labs to release a free COVID-19 care-planning guide, which provides information and actions steps for those considering their health priorities and their health-care decision-maker. General advance care planning tools are also getting more attention; in March 2020, there was a significant spike in requests for a popular end-of-life planning document called "Five Wishes" (Aleccia, 2020). States have relaxed regulations about necessary notarizations of signatures (Rosenbloom et al., 2020). Social workers can take advantage of this new energy and continue to press the importance of self-awareness, communication of preferences, and completion of legal documents in advance of illness and dying.

Social isolation

Social isolation and loneliness in older adults have long been concerns of gerontological social workers (Lubben et al., 2018). Older adults are at increased risk due to the potential for decreased mobility, sensory impairment, chronic health conditions, and smaller social networks; and it is estimated that 25% of people over the age of 65 are socially isolated, and a larger number experience loneliness (National Academies of Sciences, Engineering and Medicine, 2020). Further, negative health outcomes including depression, anxiety, cognitive decline, cardiovascular disease, and obesity have been associated with social isolation (National Academies of Sciences, Engineering and Medicine, 2020). In the current pandemic, as we stay at home and restrict social contact, the realities of isolation and loneliness are becoming clear in a new way.

In response to increased awareness, resources around social isolation and loneliness have been developed and disseminated to educate and assist people touched by these issues (Davidson, 2020; "COVID-19 free service to all new customers," 2020; Span, 2020). Creative ways to connect socially, while being physically separate, are also emerging. Older adults are using on-line platforms to visit with friends and family. There are campaigns to write letters or send cards to older adults living in facilities and programs where volunteers and older adults can virtually visit each other. This increased visibility is bringing loneliness and social isolation to the forefront in unprecedented ways. Social workers can work to ensure that routine assessments, information and referral resources, care-planning, and public health campaigns continue to focus on this important issue.

On-line connection for service provision

Despite its promise, older adults have been slow to embrace telehealth as an alternative to traditional medical care, partially explained by lack of equipment, discomfort with technology, and lack of trust that telehealth is safe and dependable ("Seniors and Telehealth," 2020). However, since the start of the pandemic, there has been rapid movement toward the on-line provision of services to protect health care workers and clients/patients from unnecessary exposure (Siwicki, 2020). Indeed, the COVID-19 outbreak caused providers across the country to build on-line infrastructure for patient use.

Due to the coronavirus, the Centers for Medicare and Medicaid Services have temporarily expanded telehealth regulations to include a number of previously uncovered services. Now, virtual visits with physicians, nurse practitioners, clinical psychologists, and clinical social workers are covered. (Robeznieks, 2020). Similarly, mHealth, which typically refers to a patient digitally tracking and reporting health information through a device or app, is a rapidly developing field ("Seniors and Telehealth," 2020). Health and social service providers have attempted to get necessary equipment to people in need and organizations are more active in teaching clients how to use these platforms (Cassata, 2020). The growth in telehealth and mHealth marks a potential shift in how healthcare services are delivered in this country; and older adults have much to gain from these technologies. Social workers must adopt these on-line strategies to provide social services, advocate for on-going reimbursement of these services, and lead efforts to ensure that all people have access to the equipment and skills that they need.

Productive engagement and intergenerational solidarity

Despite the dominant narrative that older adults are vulnerable and need to be protected during this pandemic, we need to spotlight older people who are working from home and in the essential roles where they are most exposed to infection; who continue to volunteer and find creative ways to contribute to communities; and who are caregivers to relatives and friends who may need more assistance than ever. Productive aging advocates have long pointed out that ageist attitudes and outdated social structures limit participation of older adults in these important roles (Morrow-Howell et al., 2018). We now have the opportunity to call out contributions that are being made in these most challenging of times, as well as call for increasing engagement in these vital roles as part of the recovery ahead.

To support recovery in families, communities, and the economy at large, we can argue for policy and program developments to support older people in employment, education, informal and formal caregiving, and civic engagement activities. Principles of health equity, choice, opportunity, and inclusion are forefront. A dedication to intergenerational solidarity is critical. Generational tensions are a threat, as younger people may feel that they are shouldering the economic burden to protect older people from the virus (Keating, 2020). Social workers are centrally involved in intergenerational programming; and we need to promote, spotlight, and celebrate intergenerational acts of service during this pandemic. We know that acts of intergenerational community-building are occurring across the country; and Generations United has released guides to inform socially distant intergenerational programs and activities (see https://www.gu.org). Moving forward, we would like to see the intergenerational connections that have been created during this crisis become ingrained.

Conclusion

The three gerontological social work perspectives reviewed here are familiar to social workers and pervade our research and educational agendas. The fact that they are so applicable during the coronavirus pandemic reminds us of their fundamental relevance. We can confront the ageism highlighted during the pandemic by continually reminding people of the heterogeneity of the older population. We can explain the disproportionate burden of COVID-19 on people of color and with lower socioeconomic status using concepts of cumulative disadvantage and intersectionality. These understandings can motivate efforts to reduce disparity through policy and program interventions. The strength-based perspective encourages us to seize opportunities for positive social developments. At the moment, we can build on renewed interest to expand advanced planning and reduce social isolation; and we can support older adults and providers as they embrace technology for on-line service provision. We can reject ageist discourse when it surfaces, bolster our arguments for supporting older adults as workers, volunteers, and caregivers, and actively promote efforts to expand intergenerational solidarity. Gerontological social work has much to offer in our roles as researchers, educators, practitioners and advocates during this crisis, and our fundamental principles serve us well.

References

Accius, J., & Suh, J. Y. (2019, December). *The longevity economy outlook: How people ages 50 and older are fueling economic growth, stimulating jobs, and creating opportunities for all.* AARP Thought Leadership. https://doi.org/10.26419/int.00042.001

Telehealth and seniors. (2020, April). Aging in Place. https://www.aginginplace.org/telehealth-and-seniors/

Aleccia, J. (2020, March 31). *Sheltered at home, families broach end-of-life planning.* Kaiser Health News. https://khn.org/news/coronavirus-medical-directives-end-of-life-planning/

Ault, A. (2020, April 10). *Alabama alters COVID-19 vent policy after discrimination complaints*. Medscape. https://www.medscape.com/viewarticle/928524?nlid=134997_3901&src=wnl_newsalrt_200412_MSCPEDIT&uac=324770DY&impID=2344371&faf=1

Barnes, P. (2020, March 13). *Did U.S. response to COVID-19 lag due to age discrimination?* Forbes. https://www.forbes.com/sites/patriciagbarnes/2020/03/13/did-us-response-to-covid-19-lag-due-to-age-discrimination/#3d79c1491784

Brunkard, J., Namulanda, G., & Ratard, R. (2008). Hurricane Katrina deaths, Louisiana, 2005. *Disaster Medicine and Public Health Preparedness, 2*(4), 215–223. https://doi.org/10.1097/DMP.0b013e31818aaf55

Carnethon, M., Pu, J., Howard, G., Albert, M., Anderson, C., Bertoni, A., Mujahid, M. S., Palaniappan, L., Taylor, H. A., Willis, M. & Yancy, C. (2017). Cardiovascular health in African Americans: A scientific statement from the American Heart Association. *American Heart Association Journal, 136*(21), e393–e423. https://doi.org/10.1161/CIR.0000000000000534

Cassata, C. (2020 April 15). *Why a virtual visit to the doctor may be the safest, most affordable option*. Healthline. https://www.healthline.com/health-news/telehealth-and-covid-19

Chen, E. (2020, March 31). *As nursing homes struggle with coronavirus prevention, residents become more isolated*. St. Louis Public Radio. https://news.stlpublicradio.org/post/nursing-homes-struggle-coronavirus-prevention-residents-become-more-isolated#stream/0

Coughlin, J., & Yoquinto, L. (2020, April 13). Many parts of America have already decided to sacrifice the elderly. *The Washington Post*. https://www.washingtonpost.com/outlook/2020/04/13/many-parts-america-have-already-decided-sacrifice-elderly/

COVID-19 free service for all new customers. (2020, March 16). Iamfine. https://dailycall.iamfine.com/covid-19/

Davidson, J. (2020, April 23). *Isolation: The hidden risk of social distancing*. Everyday Health. https://www.everydayhealth.com/coronavirus/isolation-the-hidden-risk-of-social-distancing/

Dosa, D., Feng, Z., Hyer, K., Brown, L. M., Thomas, K., & Mor, V. (2010). Effects of Hurricane Katrina on nursing facility resident mortality, hospitalization, and functional decline. *Disaster Medicine and Public Health Preparedness, 4*(Suppl 1(0 1)), S28–S32. https://doi.org/10.1001/dmp.2010.11

Family Caregiver Alliance. (2019, April 17). *Caregiver Statistics: Demographics*. National Center on Caregiving. https://www.caregiver.org/caregiver-statistics-demographics

Hamel, L. W. (2017, April 27). *Views and experiences with end-of-life medical care in the U.S.* Kaiser Family Foundation. https://www.kff.org/other/report/views-and-experiences-with-end-of-life-medical-care-in-the-u-s/

Hargrave, R. (2010). *Health and health care of African American older adults*. eCampus Geriatrics. https://geriatrics.stanford.edu/wp-content/uploads/2014/10/african_american.pdf

Health benefits of senior corps. (2018, August). Corporation for National and Community Service https://www.nationalservice.gov/sites/default/files/documents/IssueBrief-Health-Benefits-of-Senior-Corps-02052019_508_0.pdf

Keating, J. (2020, April, 14). *The coronavirus recovery could pit the old and young against each other*. Slate. https://slate.com/news-and-politics/2020/04/graying-populations-economic-recovery.html

Klinenberg, E. (2002). *Heat wave: a social autopsy of disaster in Chicago*. Chicago University Press.

Kurtzleben, D. (2020, April 22). *Job losses higher among people of color during the coronavirus pandemic*. National Public Radio. https://www.npr.org/2020/04/22/840276956/minorities-often-work-these-jobs-they-were-among-first-to-go-in-coronavirus-layo

Liska, L. (2020, April 6). *Senior volunteers sew cloth masks to help prevent the spread of COVID-19.* WLTZ First News. https://www.wltz.com/2020/04/06/sewing-masks-sew-cloth-masks-to-help-prevent-the-spread-of-covid-19/

Lowsky, D. O. (2014). Heterogeneity in healthy aging. *The Journals of Gerontology Series A: Biological and Medical Sciences, 69*(6), 640–649. https://doi.org/10.1093/gerona/glt162

Lubben, J. E., Tracy, E., Crewe, S. E., Sabbath, E., Gironda, M., Johnson, C., Kong, J., Munson, M., & Brown, S. (2018). Eradicate social isolation. In R. Fong, J. Lubben, & R. P. Barth (Eds.), *Grand challenges for social work and society.* (pp. 103-123). Oxford University Press.

Maqbool, A. (2020, April 11). *Coronavirus: Why has the virus hit African-Americans so hard?* BBC News. https://www.bbc.com/news/world-us-canada-52245690

Markowitz, A. (2020, March 25). *AARP community connections offers ways to find help.* AARP. https://www.aarp.org/politics-society/advocacy/info-2020/aarp-community-connections.html?cmp=SNO-ABC-FB-COVID-LC&socialid=3284494125

Miller, R. (2020, March 27). *101-year-old Italian man, born amid Spanish flu pandemic, survives coronavirus illness, official says.* USA Today. https://www.usatoday.com/story/news/world/2020/03/27/italy-101-year-old-born-during-spanish-flu-survives-coronavirus/2926073001/

Morath, E., & Feintzeig, R. (2020, March 20). *'I have bills I have to pay.' Low-wage workers face brunt of coronavirus crisis.* Wall Street Journal. https://www.wsj.com/articles/i-have-bills-i-have-to-pay-low-wage-workers-face-brunt-of-coronavirus-crisis-11584719927

Morrow-Howell, N., Gonzales, E., James, J., Matz-Costa, C., & Putnam, M. (2018). Advancing long and productive lives. In R. Fong, J. Lubben, & R. Barth (Eds.), *Grand challenges for social work and society.* (pp. 81-102). Oxford University Press.

National Academies of Sciences, Engineering, and Medicine. (2020). *Social isolation and loneliness in older adults: Opportunities for the health care system.* The National Academies Press.

National Association of Social Workers Delegate Assembly. (2017). *Code of ethics of the national association of social workers.* NASW Press.

Reid, A. (2020, April 6). *Coronavirus Philadelphia: Positive tests higher in poorer neighborhoods despite six times more testing in higher-income neighborhoods, researcher says.* CBS Philly. https://philadelphia.cbslocal.com/2020/04/06/coronavirus-philadelphia-positive-tests-higher-in-poorer-neighborhoods-despite-six-times-more-testing-in-higher-income-neighborhoods-researcher-says/

Robeznieks, A. (2020, March 19). *Key changes made to telehealth guidelines to boost COVID-19 care.* American Medical Association. https://www.ama-assn.org/delivering-care/public-health/key-changes-made-telehealth-guidelines-boost-covid-19-care

Rosenbloom, A., Matz, K., Brandman, E., Herzberg, S., & Martinez, D. (2020, April 8). *'Virtual Witnessing' of wills, lifetime trusts, health care proxies, and durable powers of attorney is allowed in New York state through May 7, 2020.* Stroock. https://www.stroock.com/publication/virtual-witnessing-of-wills-lifetime-trusts-health-care-proxies-and-durable-powers-of-attorney-is-allowed-in-new-york-state-through-may-7-2020/

Siwicki, B. (2020, March 19). *Telemedicine during COVID-19: Benefits, limitations, burdens, adaptation.* Healthcare IT News. https://www.healthcareitnews.com/news/telemedicine-during-covid-19-benefits-limitations-burdens-adaptation=

Sohn, H. (2017). Racial and ethnic disparities in health insurance coverage: Dynamics of gaining and losing coverage over the life-course. *Population Research and Policy Review, 36*(2), 181–201. https://doi.org/10.1007/s11113-016-9416-y

Sonmez, F. (2020, March 24). Texas Lt. Gov. Dan Patrick comes under fire for saying seniors should 'take a chance' on their own lives for sake of grandchildren during coronavirus crisis. *The Washington Post.* https://www.washingtonpost.com/politics/texas-lt-gov-dan-patrick-comes-under-fire-for-saying-seniors-should-take-a-chance-on-their-own-lives-for-sake-of-grandchildren-during-coronavirus-crisis/2020/03/24/e6f64858-6de6-11ea-b148-e4ce3fbd85b5_story.html

Span, P. (2020, April 13). *Just what older people didn't need: More isolation.* The New York Times. https://www.nytimes.com/2020/04/13/health/coronavirus-elderly-isolation-loneliness.html?fbclid=IwAR1dLpzQ80aXG8ERacNtMvfkej01IOBX3nKEJO72MEEmwkacvLQxfODqKP0

Taylor, K. (2020, April 16). *The black plague.* The New Yorker. https://www.newyorker.com/news/our-columnists/the-black-plague?link_id=5&can_id=28d1aa70d5b5aa1fdf493c8cd6b2a398&source=email-racism-is-a-public-health-issue-cancelrent-global-covid-19-solidarity&email_referrer=email_784489&email_subject=covid19-racial-justice-from-cancel-rent-to-clts-sharemycheck

The Eisner Foundation. (2020, March 23). *COVID-19: How our partners are adapting.* https://eisnerfoundation.org/eisner-journal/covid-19-how-our-partners-are-adapting/

U.S. Bureau of Labor Statistics. (n.d.). *U.S. labor force shares by age, 1970 to 2014 and projected 2014–24.* Bureau of Labor Statistics. https://www.bls.gov/careeroutlook/2017/article/older-workers.htm

COVID-19 Pandemic: Workforce Implications for Gerontological Social Work

Marla Berg-Weger and Tracy Schroepfer

ABSTRACT

The COVID-19 pandemic has been challenging for people of all ages but particularly devastating to adults 65 and older, which has highlighted the critical need for ensuring that all social workers gain the knowledge and skills necessary to work with this population. While there is a critical shortage of gerontological social workers and we must continue to increase that number, we cannot wait for this to occur. In this commentary, the authors call for infusing the current social work curricula with aging content; providing current social workers with trainings on aging practice; and all social work practitioners, faculty, and researchers to address four specific areas that have gained prominence due to the impact of COVID-19: ageism, loneliness and social isolation, technology, and interprofessional practice, in their respective areas.

The COVID-19 pandemic has been challenging for people of all ages but particularly devastating to adults 65 and older. In the United States, 4,226 cases were reported between February 12 and March 16. Of these cases, older adults comprised 31% of cases, 45% of hospitalizations, 53% of ICU admissions, and 80% of deaths (CDC COVID-19 Response Team, 2020). Accordingly, the CDC has raised concerns regarding the increase in services necessary to support older adults and their families. Many of these services will require the assistance of gerontological social workers, who are trained to work in the area of aging.

We have long known of a social worker shortage, particularly in gerontological social work. Wang and Chonody (2013) reported that only 1,000 students were annually specializing in gerontological social work, while 5,000 additional gerontologically-trained social workers were needed to meet the needs of older adults in practice. The COVID-19 pandemic, however, has increased the need for even greater numbers of gerontological social workers. These social work practitioners have been on the frontlines of this crisis supporting older adults, their families, and the professionals who provide care and services. In addition, gerontological social work scholars have been providing education/training to professionals, students, and the community; publishing necessary information and guidance; and conducting research projects to better understand the ways in which the pandemic is impacting practice with older adults. Whether in the field or the virtual classroom, gerontological practitioners and scholars have demonstrated their knowledge, skills, and values; however, it is apparent that the shortage of these skilled social workers is critical.

The social work profession takes pride in its history of responding to societal needs and while our social work knowledge, skills, and values prepare us well to respond to the current pandemic, the lack of social workers trained to work with older adults is problematic. Although we should not lose focus on increasing the number of gerontological social workers, it is crucial that we recognize the urgency of the current situation and begin making key changes now. For our current and future social work students, Schools of Social Work must look to infuse aging content across the curriculum such that all students graduate with the knowledge and skills necessary to work effectively with older adults. Trainings focused on aging must also be made available to those social work practitioners who do not possess this knowledge and skills. How long this pandemic will last and the impacts it will have on current and future older adults is not yet fully known; however, current numbers from the CDC provide sufficient evidence that the dire need for social workers trained to work with this population will continue well into the future

So, where do we begin? We begin by encouraging those providing education and training to current and future social workers to review curricula and training content to ensure that it provides a foundation of aging-related knowledge and skills. Four particular areas that have emerged and gained prominence since the COVID-19 pandemic began: ageism, technology/tele-health, loneliness and social isolation, and interprofessional practice.

Ageism

Ageism has been sadly and frequently demonstrated throughout the pandemic, including lack of protocols for older adults, lack of geriatric-specific content in the curricula of the helping professions caring for older adults, inequities in allocation of needed resources, disparaging references made about COVID-19 and older adults (e.g., "Boomer remover") and relief that it is the older adults who are dying (Aronson, 2020; Cesari & Proietti, 2020). Ayalon and colleagues (2020) urge professionals in the helping professions to stress the risk factors (e.g., chronic conditions) and the impact of social distancing that promote the "digital divide" for many older adults. We must educate current and future social workers on how to confront ageist attitudes and practices and advocate for change at the micro, mezzo and macro levels.

Technology/Telehealth

While the use of technology is not a new resource for teaching, practicing, and researching gerontological social work, technology is leaving an indelible mark on the way in which our society has survived during the pandemic. Along with our students, colleagues, providers, and clients, we have used technology to teach, learn, and educate; provide services; and stay connected professionally and personally. What are we including in our curricula and research about incorporating technology into practice and research, particularly with older adults? Are we teaching students to practically and ethically deliver services, including group facilitation via telehealth platforms and how to integrate artificial intelligence into practice? Are we writing about innovative ways to intervene (e.g., using 3D printed objects for reminiscence with older adults with dementia) and researching the effectiveness of tele-delivered services (e.g., online group intervention for older adults and their caregivers)? These are the questions social work educators must answer by infusing necessary knowledge and practice skills within the curriculum.

Loneliness and social isolation

Loneliness and social isolation is not a new concern for older adults; however, the pandemic has brought broader awareness about the risks and conse-quences for all age groups and older adults, in particular (Berg-Weger & Morley, 2020a, b). Experiencing loneliness and/or social isolation can nega-tively impact myriad issues, including: physical health, including cardiovas-cular health (Molloy et al., 2010; Valtorta et al., 2016); cognitive function (Cacioppo & Cacioppo, 2014); mental health (i.e., depression) (Kabátová et al., 2016); and quality-of-life (Jakobsson & Hallberg, 2005). Outcomes associated with chronic loneliness and social isolation (longer than four years) include such conditions as hypertension, weight gain, smoking/sub-stance use, stroke, heart disease, and alone time (Cigna, 2018; Valtorta et al., 2016). As educators and practitioners, we can address these issues by including loneliness and social isolation into the assessment and intervention strategies delivered in coursework and continuing education. As researchers, we can study risk factors and prevention strategies, evaluate existing individual and group interventions, and test innovative interventions (e.g., use of technology).

Interprofessional practice

The pandemic is challenging the traditional ways in which professionals communicate and work with one another interprofessionally in institutional and community settings. The Council on Social Work Education (CSWE) has recognized the importance of training social workers with the skills necessary to work effectively with other professionals. In 2016, CSWE became an institutional member of the Interprofessional Education Collaborative (IPEC), whose mission is to "ensure that new and current health professionals are proficient in the competencies essential for patient-centered, community and population oriented, interprofessional, collaborative practice" (Council on Social Work Education, 2016). In 2018, CSWE hosted the Interprofessional Education Summit at its Annual Program Meeting with the goal of gathering together leaders and educators seeking to strengthen interprofessional practice among social workers (Council on Social Work Education, 2018). Although CSWE recognizes the importance of interprofessional education, this pandemic calls on the profession to review our approaches to interprofessional education, practice, and research, and to strengthen and supplement where necessary. We should determine if the current strategies are effective and adapt as needed those for future implementation.

Next steps

To promote gerontological social work and the infusion of aging content throughout the social work curriculum, funding is critical for students, faculty, practitioners, and researchers. Many of us benefitted from the support provided through the John A. Hartford Foundation whose goal was to increase the geriatric component of social work education to meet the demands of an aging society (John A. Hartford Foundation, 2019). Through this support, we began taking the steps necessary to integrate gerontology content into curricula, provide aging-focused practicum experiences for students and field instructors, and gain professional development experience in teaching and research. Now, we must advocate for resources that would enable us to again focus programming on curricular- and profession-wide initiatives such that social workers are prepared with the skills and training they need to work with older adults during this pandemic and after. An example of one such program is the Health Resources and Services Administration Geriatric Workforce Enhancement Program funding emphasizes interprofessional, aging-focused education and training for all students and professionals who work with older adults. More programs like this are essential if we are to promote the development of gerontology majors and minors at the undergraduate level; expand gerontology certificates, specializations, and concentrations at the graduate level to include an interprofessional perspective; and work with university development offices to develop endowments and scholarships in aging. These strategies are essential for ensuring that Schools of Social Work across the nation are graduating alumni who are prepared to practice with older adults. As many social work programs are experiencing the retirement of senior faculty, we also need funding that increase the number of well-trained social work scholars who can educate our students and conduct research in gerontological social work. The Association for Gerontology Education in Social Work Pre-Dissertation Fellows Initiative is an example of a program that has been shown to be effective in supporting doctoral students committed to gerontological social work academic careers (Schroepfer et al., 2020).

Conclusion

While the COVID-19 pandemic of 2020 will be remembered as a global crisis unlike any in recent history, we will all gain information and skills that will change our personal and professional lives beyond becoming experts in videoconferencing. As gerontological social work educators, practitioners and researchers, we must work to ensure that our social work workforce has the education and training necessary to meet the demands that COVID-19 has placed on us. We must commit to providing the best care possible to older adults and their families impacted by COVID-19 both now and post-pandemic. Together, let us use this experience to bring forward the innovations that are being developed in this time of crisis and fight for the needs of our profession, students and, most importantly, the older adults who have given so much for our nation.

Disclosures

The authors declare there are no conflicts

References

Aronson, L. (2020). *Ageism is making pandemic worse. The Atlantic.* Retrieved from: https://www.theatlantic.com/culture/archive/2020/03/americas-ageism-crisis-is-helping-the-coronavirus/608905/

Ayalon, L., Chasteen, A., Diehl, M., Levy, B., Neupert, S. D., Rothermund, K., Tesch-Römer, C., & Wahl, H. W. (2020). Aging in times of the COVID-19 pandemic: Avoid ageism and fostering intergenerational solidarity. *Journal of Gerontology, Epub Ahead of Print.* Epub ahead of print. https://doi.org/10.1093/geronb/gbaa051

Berg-Weger, M., & Morley, J. E. (2020a). Loneliness and social Isolation in older adults during the COVID-19 pandemic: Implications for gerontological social work. *Journal of Nutrition, Health, & Aging, 24*(5), 456–458. https://doi.org/10.1007/s12603-020-1366-8

Cacioppo, J. T., & Cacioppo, S. (2014). Older adults reporting social isolation or loneliness show poorer cognitive function 4 years later. *Evidence-Based Nursing, 17*(2), 59–60. https://doi.org/10.1136/eb-2013-101379

CDC COVID-19 Response Team. (2020). Severe outcomes among patients with coronavirus disease 2019 (COVID-19) — United States, February 12–March 16. *MMWR Morbidity Morality Weekly Report, 69*(12), 343–346. https://doi.org/http://dx.doi.10.15585/mmwr.mm6912e2externalicon

Cesari, M., & Proietti, M. (2020). Geriatric medicine in Italy in the time of COVID-19. *Journal of Nutrition, Health, and Aging, 24*, 1–2. https://doi.org/10.1007/s12603-020-1354-z

Cigna. (2018). *Cigna U.S. loneliness index.* Cigna. Retrieved from: https://www.cigna.com/assets/docs/newsroom/loneliness-survye-2018-fact-sheet.pdf

Council on Social Work Education. (2016). *CSWE among newest members of interprofessional education collaborative.* Council on Social Work Education. Retrieved from: https://www.cswe.org/News/Press-Room/Press-Release-Archives/CSWE-Among-Newest-Members-of-Interprofessional-EduEdu

Council on Social Work Education. (2018). *Interprofessional Education Summit.* Council on Social Work Education. Retrieved from: https://www.cswe.org/Events-Meetings/APM-Archives/2018-APM/Conference-Program/Post-conference-Interprofessional-Education-Summit

Jakobsson, U., & Hallberg, I. R. (2005). Loneliness, fear, and quality of life among elderly in Sweden: A gender perspective. *Aging Clinical and Experimental Research, 17*(6), 494–501. https://doi.org/10.1007/BF03327417

John, A. (2019). Assessment of the accomplishments and impact of the John A. Hartford Foundation's grantmaking in aging and health 1983-1025. New York: The John A. Hartford Foundation. Retrieved from: https://www.johnahartford.org/images/uploads/reports/JAHF_Accomplishments_Impact_Report_FINAL_1.7.2019.pdf

Kabátová, O., Puteková, S., & Martinková, J. (2016). Loneliness as a risk factor for depression in the elderly. *Clinical Social Work, 7*(1), 48-52. DOI: 10.22359/cswhi_7_1_05

Molloy, G. J., McGee, H. M., O'Neill, D., & Conroy, R. M. (2010). Loneliness and emergency and planned hospitalizations in a community sample of older adults. *Journal of the American Geriatrics Society, 58*(8), 1538–1541. https://doi.org/10.1111/j.1532-5415.2010.02960.x

Schroepfer, T., Berg-Weger, M., & Morano, C. (2020). Training the next generation of gerontological social work scholars. *Journal of Gerontological Social Work, 62*(8), 823–827. https://doi.org/10.1080/01634372.2019.1663461

Valtorta, N. K., Kanaan, M., Gilbody, S., Ronzi, S., & Hanratty, B. (2016). Loneliness and social isolation as risk factors for coronary heart disease and stroke: Systematic review and meta-analysis of longitudinal observational studies. *Heart, 102*(13), 1009–1016. https://doi.org/10.1136/heartjnl-2015-308790

Wang, D., & Chonody, J. (2013). Social workers' attitudes toward older adults: A review of the literature. *Journal of Social Work Education, 49*(1), 150–172. https://doi.org/10.1080/10437797.2013.755104

Older Workers in the Time of COVID-19: The Senior Community Service Employment Program and Implications for Social Work

Cal J. Halvorsen ⓘD and Olga Yulikova

ABSTRACT

It has long been the goal of many gerontological social work scholars to increase the ability and opportunity for people to be engaged in paid and unpaid work throughout the life course. Yet the COVID-19 pandemic is revealing and exacerbating the financial insecurity of many older adults. In this paper, we review information related to older workers and how they might be affected by this pandemic and its aftermath, paying particular attention to the most socioeconomically and physically vulnerable older workers. We also offer first-hand experiences from our careers working with and conducting scholarship on older workers, paying particular attention to recent actions by many in the Senior Community Service Employment Program (SCSEP) network to provide paid sick leave to its low-income, older adult participants. We conclude with implications for social work scholarship and teaching, noting the uptick in technology use among older adults and the disparities that remain, as well as teaching that integrates discussions on the lifelong and cumulative effects of inequalities and marginalization and the need for additional researcher, student, and community collaborations.

Introduction

Increasing the ability and opportunity for people to stay economically, civically, and socially engaged throughout the lifespan are important aspects of the Grand Challenges for Social Work initiative (see Lubben et al., 2015; Morrow-Howell et al., 2015). And through the novel coronavirus pandemic, these challenges have become both increasingly apparent and, often, severe.

In this paper, we review information related to older workers and how they might be affected by this pandemic and its aftermath, paying particular attention to the most economically and physically vulnerable older workers. We also offer first-hand experiences from our careers working with and conducting scholarship on older workers, highlighting the recent actions by many grantees in the Senior Community Service Employment Program (SCSEP) network to provide paid sick leave to the program's low-income, older adult participants. We conclude with implications for program operators and gerontological social workers regarding technology use among financially vulnerable older adults, social work scholarship and teaching that integrates concepts of cumulative disadvantage, and a call for social work scholars to pursue additional collaborations with aging services providers and older adults themselves.

Older workers in an aging America

The U.S. is rapidly aging. In fact, 2019 was the first year that the U.S. had more people over the age of 60 than under the age of 18 (Halvorsen, 2019). While older Americans are, by and large, healthier than previous generations – death rates for heart disease, cancer, and stroke have declined among those older than 65 since 2000 (National Center for Health Statistics, 2018) – these gains have been unequal, including for black and Hispanic populations (see, for example, Centers for Disease Control and Prevention, 2013). We also know that this growing aging population is more susceptible than younger people to the worst effects of COVID-19, the disease caused by the novel coronavirus, SARS-CoV-2, especially for those with preexisting medical conditions like heart or lung disease or diabetes (Centers for Disease Control and Prevention, 2020). Further, older adults of color and those who have lower socioeconomic status face higher levels of risk, both physically from the virus and financially from the economic fallout (Morrow-Howell et al., 2020).

Well before this pandemic, gerontological social work scholars have documented the needs and desires for people in later life to work longer, as well as their experiences in doing so, in volunteer and pro-bono roles (Morrow-Howell, 2010; Pitt-Catsouphes et al., 2017), as wage or salary workers (Choi et al., 2018; Morrow-Howell et al., 2017), in self-employment (Halvorsen & Chen, 2019; Halvorsen & Morrow-Howell, 2017), and in "encores" for the social good in new careers and as social entrepreneurs (Halvorsen & Chen, 2019; Halvorsen & Emerman, 2014).

Yet in our careers focused on making it easier for older people to seek paid work – the first author formerly in the private sector at the national nonprofit organization, Encore.org, and now in academia at Boston College; and the coauthor, the Massachusetts state director of the Senior Community Service Employment Program – we know that the effects of cumulative advantage and disadvantage are real and supported by empirical data (e.g., Crystal et al., 2017; Dingemans et al., 2016). The effects of cumulative advantage due to discrimination and marginalization across the life course in areas such as education, employment, housing, health care, and more are already being displayed through this pandemic (Swinford et al., 2020). Further, older workers are finding it harder to continue working and often lack key benefits that could keep them, their coworkers, and their families safe, such as remote working arrangements and paid sick leave (Alwin & Schramm, 2020; Gould, 2020).

Finding and keeping work in later life was difficult before this pandemic and most certainly is now. During the recession after 2008, for example, the length of time spent receiving unemployment benefits increased dramatically for workers aged 62 and older (Johnson, 2012). Further, older workers face a decent chance of losing their jobs even during good economic times: More than half of full-time, full-year workers in their early 50s with a long-term employer have been shown to be involuntarily separated from their jobs (Johnson & Gosselin, 2018), with clear racial and ethnic differences in factors associated with working longer that highlight the relative advantage of older white Americans (Choi et al., 2017). In the years just prior to the start of this pandemic, nearly three in four workers aged 65 and older could not work from home (Gould, 2020); in today's context, this inability to work remotely may force many older workers to put themselves at physical risk to continue to earn an income. And in a harbinger of what may come, important stakeholders, including the U.S. Chamber of Commerce, have floated the idea of allowing organizations to bar older workers from returning to the workplace due to concerns that they would be more vulnerable to COVID-19 (Tankersley & Savage, 2020). Without important protections and safety nets, the physical and financial consequences of this pandemic are and will continue to be far-reaching for older workers.

As such, our society faces a conundrum for older workers and other groups of people more vulnerable to the effects of COVID-19: heightened risk of physical harm or death for returning to work yet financial devastation for not doing so. These risks might be further enhanced for workers not eligible for Medicare (typically those under the age of 65; see U.S. Department of Health & Human Services, 2014), which is covering lab tests and antibody tests with no out-of-pocket costs, as well as medically necessary hospitalizations for COVID-19 at the standard rates (U.S. Centers for Medicare & Medicaid Services, 2020).

Continuing benefits for older workers within the Senior Community Service Employment Program

One particularly vulnerable group of older workers are those who take part in the Senior Community Service Employment Program (SCSEP), a federal program authorized by Title V of the Older Americans Act of 1965 that acts as both an anti-poverty and workforce training program for people aged 55 and older who are unemployed, face barriers to employment, and live at or below 125% of the federal poverty level (Halvorsen & Yulikova, 2020; U.S. Department of Labor, Employment & Training Administration, 2018b). The approximately 67,000 participants in this program are paid the prevailing minimum wage at nonprofit or public organizations ("host agencies") while receiving job skills training (Halvorsen & Yulikova, 2020; Mikelson, 2017). Scholars have found that SCSEP leads to post-program unsubsidized work that pays more than they original received from the federal government (Mikelson, 2017) and that participation is linked to perceptions of better physical and mental health, social connections, self-esteem, and work skills, among others (Aday & Kehoe, 2008; Gonzales et al., 2020; U.S. Department of Labor, Employment & Training Administration, 2018a). This program is also under threat to be cut by the federal government (Halvorsen & Yulikova, 2020).

SCSEP participants are particularly vulnerable to the implications of living near or below the poverty level. They are more likely to be people of color (U.S. Department of Labor, Employment & Training Administration, 2018a, 2019), and are often reflective of unique regional diversities. In Massachusetts, for example, SCSEP participants include immigrants from Haiti, Cape Verde, and other countries. Overall, this program engages participants' motivations to find work with part-time, on-the-job training and continued income, with participants describing SCSEP as a "blessing" (Halvorsen & Yulikova, 2020) and a "lifeline" (Gonzales et al., 2020).

Many within SCSEP are expressing concerns for how this pandemic will affect the program and its participants. Some SCSEP participants have voiced their concerns over returning to work and becoming an unnecessary burden or even a liability to their host agencies; likewise, grantees have expressed concerns with keeping their older workers safe. From the grantees' perspective, the costs and logistics of workers compensation insurance might soon become an issue. Adding further complication is the fact that key program performance outcomes, including the number of hours that participants work (called "community service hours") and their earnings in unsubsidized employment after leaving SCSEP, will be dramatically reduced (e.g., U.S. Department of Labor, Employment & Training Administration, 2018c). Encouragingly, the Department of Labor has been a proactive and receptive administrator, listening to grantees about the challenges that they, their host agencies, and their participants are experiencing today. This open dialogue between the federal government and state and national grantees is a helpful approach during this pandemic with multiple unknowns.

Yet in the face of this pandemic and the stay-at-home advisories in most states, it became difficult, if not impossible, for SCSEP participants to work, alarming the participants, host agencies, and grantees. Further, the process for getting to work became daunting for the many participants who rely on public transportation, especially in urban areas. And given the severe financial constraints that participants already faced, not receiving the associated income from their missed work would likely lead to a cascading influx of repercussions related to food and nutrition, housing and utilities, physical and mental health, and other factors.

As such, by the end of March 2020, many SCSEP grantees across the nation decided to continue payments to participants while temporarily suspending their work assignments through the provision of paid sick leave. This answers a key call of this program to reduce the most severe effects of poverty while temporarily freezing its second purpose, workforce training. Paid sick leave enables participants to remain at home and reduce their risk of exposure to the novel coronavirus and is allowable under guidance from the Department of Labor (U.S. Department of Labor, Employment & Training Administration, 2020). Note that SCSEP funding is distributed among a diverse set of 19 national nonprofit and 56 state and territorial grantees, and each program may be facing different sets of circumstances that influence their ability to take similar actions.

This is a temporary solution, providing a patch in a precariously strung-together social safety net that requires bold solutions at multiple levels. *Yet it is a start.* As the economy begins to open, the SCSEP network will work with host agencies and participants to determine the smartest approach to reintegrating participants in the workplace, whether that be a return to the physical workplace or remote work when possible. Participants have also been invited – but not required – to engage in online job skills training programs while home. This takes into account the variability in participants' access to fast and affordable internet as well as computers or smartphones. Many participants, for example, rely on flip phones with limited minutes and data or landlines.

Implications for social work

This pandemic, through its unearthing of severe issues related to financially insecure older adults, is revealing important implications for social work scholars and teachers.

Older adults are more technologically savvy and connected than stereotypes suggest – yet disparities still exist by age and income

While it may feel opportunistic to focus on the positives related to this pandemic, we do want to focus on some good news. Just as Morrow-Howell et al. (2020) discussed, older adults are much more technologically savvy than in the near past. Due to financial and other constraints, we know that SCSEP participants have historically struggled to stay technologically connected and often had little to no access to fast internet speeds or affordable data plans. This is due partly to disparities in technological use by age, in that younger people have more online access (Vogels, 2019); by income, in that those with higher levels of income have more online access (Anderson & Kumar, 2019); and by race and ethnicity, in that white, non-Hispanic respondents are more likely to have access to computers or high-speed internet at home (Perrin &

Turner, 2019). Yet access to smartphones, tablet computers, and social media have steadily increased among older generations (Vogels, 2019), and smartphones are helping to reduce this disparity in internet access for black and Hispanic Americans (Perrin & Turner, 2019). And since the stay-at-home advisories have taken effect in many states, we have seen first-hand how many older adults – including SCSEP participants – have stayed connected online through e-mail and virtual Zoom meetings. In Massachusetts, for example, some technologically savvy SCSEP participants are helping their peers to get online, too. This is important, as many participants, who may have relied on their children or grandchildren in the past to teach them new technologies, can no longer rely on them for fear of spreading or contracting the novel coronavirus.

Yet this is not true for all participants. Many are facing major difficulties in getting online, preventing them from socially engaging with others and making it difficult for SCSEP grantees to plan future virtual trainings and meetings. One step some grantees have taken is to plan "old school" teleconference meetings instead of Zoom meetings, as well as to provide call-in numbers for virtual meetings for those who lack fast or stable internet access or webcams to stream video. Considering the larger issue, we should also rekindle discussions on how to bring fast and affordable internet access to those who need it while training newcomers to computer, tablet, or smart phone technologies in their use.

Social work scholars and teachers must stress the cumulative effects of inequalities and disadvantages from the clinical to macro levels

The financial difficulties faced by so many older workers highlights the need for social work scholars to conduct more research on and teach about work and economic insecurity among a diverse set of populations throughout the lifespan. Indeed, many of us are already doing this, yet it can be so easy to focus simply on the *effects* of inequalities and disadvantages at older ages that the often earlier-in-life and cumulative *causes* of these effects are not considered. For example, how might we, as gerontological social workers, engage with faculty and students in the children and families concentrations to study the lifelong effects of early-life influences, such as trauma, on physical, mental, and financial well-being? One resource that the first author shares when introducing this concept in his classes is the "Two Lives of Jasmine" video, created in partnership between the St. Louis PBS affiliate, Nine Network, and the For the Sake of All initiative (see Health Equity Works, 2014).

In the classroom, we can also lead discussions on clinical-macro connections that are informed by lifespan perspectives. This can bridge what can so often feel like a clear divide between students' concentrations that are not reflected in the work that many social workers actually perform at multiple levels within the system through both formal and informal tasks. Many of the frameworks that are key to the social work profession – ecological systems theory (Bronfenbrenner, 1993) and person-in-environment (Kondrat, 2002) are just two examples – stress this, yet the dichotomy continues to exist. Case studies that involve financially insecure older workers can be especially illustrative of the clinical-macro connections for students (for an example, see Halvorsen & Skees, 2019). The financial distress that so many people past midlife experience is often a result of family and community experiences, programs, and policies from earlier in life, and both clinical *and* local, state, national, organizational, and cultural interventions – often grouped together as "macro" – can work in a complementary fashion to improve the living situations for individuals and their families. The financial security of older people is certainly relevant to the future work of students interested in working with children, as many of the children they serve will be living in inter-generational households, often with grandparents serving as the primary caregivers, or nearby grandparents serving as sources of support during emergencies (Davis et al., 2020; Yancura, 2013). Indeed, an estimated one in five (20%) Americans lived in multigenerational households in 2016, up from 12% in 1980, and those from racial and ethnic minorities are more likely to live in these households than non-Hispanic white Americans (Cohn & Passel, 2018).

Gerontological social work scholars must continue to engage with community stakeholders

Those of us who study economic, civic, and social engagement in later life must continue to strengthen our focus on creating community-research partnerships with aging services providers and a diverse group of older adults themselves (e.g., Fortuna et al., 2019; Zendell et al., 2007). These are examples of public scholarship, a long-held guidepost within social work research that has received renewed recent attention and involves reciprocal exchanges of information and conversations between scholars and the community in research, teaching, and service with a goal of reaching and supporting marginalized groups (for an in-depth discussion, see Sliva et al., 2019). This pandemic is only increasing the need for public scholarship. The authors of this paper, for example, have started to engage in public-private collaborations with the aim of strengthening SCSEP (e.g., Halvorsen & Yulikova, 2020). Future plans include to document the experiences of SCSEP participants among a range of antecedents and outcomes at the individual, organizational, and community levels, as well as to use participants' and case managers' own voices to shape program and policy recommendations to strengthen SCSEP.

Conclusion

It has long been the goal of many gerontological social work scholars to increase the ability and opportunity to be engaged in paid and unpaid work throughout the lifespan. Yet COVID-19 is both revealing and exacerbating the financial insecurity faced by many older people as well as highlighting the increased physical vulnerabilities of older workers. In this article, we reviewed some of the literature on the needs of older workers and gave a first-hand account of how many in the Senior Community Service Employment Program network are responding to this crisis to benefit participants, including through the provision of paid sick leave. We concluded with implications for social work scholarship and teaching, noting the uptick in technology use among older adults and the disparities that may remain, as well as the lifelong and cumulative effects of inequalities and marginalization and the need for additional researcher, student, and community collaborations.

We end with some anecdotes of Massachusetts SCSEP participants that highlight the desire for continued economic, civic, and social engagement of lower-income, older workers. One participant spoke of the loss of a sense of meaning in her life due to the loss of her work. Another participant spoke of his desire to get back to work and simultaneous fear of exposure to the novel coronavirus due to his need to take four buses to get to work. Many are finding ways to give back to their communities when sheltering at home. A team of two participants contacted their peers in the program to help them learn how to use Zoom and other technologies to stay connected. Another participant started sewing cloth face masks to give to essential workers for free. And a former participant joined the efforts of Massachusetts and the nonprofit organization, Partners in Health, by becoming a contact tracer (see Massachusetts Executive Office of Health and Human Services, 2020).

While the pandemic caused by the novel coronavirus has dramatically slowed our economy and temporarily kept most people at home – including SCSEP participants and other older workers – we know that many older people both need and want to work. Moving forward, gerontological social workers must take part in conversations to maintain and increase opportunities for older workers, especially lower-income older workers, to stay economically, civically, and socially engaged in their communities.

Disclosure statement

Olga Yulikova, MA, has directed the Senior Community Service Employment Program in the Massachusetts Executive Office of Elder Affairs for more than 11 years. Arguments in this manuscript represent her personal views and do not represent the official positions of her program or employer. Cal J. Halvorsen declares no conflict of interest.

Funding

The authors declare no sources of funding for this work.

ORCID

Cal J. Halvorsen (iD) http://orcid.org/0000-0002-9184-633X

References

Aday, R. H., & Kehoe, G. (2008). Working in old age: Benefits of participation in the senior community service employment program. *Journal of Workplace Behavioral Health*, *23*(1–2), 125–145. https://doi.org/10.1080/15555240802189521

Alwin, R. L., & Schramm, J. (2020, April 3). *Coronavirus' economic impact on older workers. AARP.* http://www.aarp.org/politics-society/advocacy/info-2020/coronavirus-economic-impact-older-workers.html

Anderson, M., & Kumar, M. (2019). *Digital divide persists even as lower-income Americans make gains in tech adoption.* Pew Research Center. https://www.pewresearch.org/fact-tank/2019/05/07/digital-divide-persists-even-as-lower-income-americans-make-gains-in-tech-adoption/

Bronfenbrenner, U. (1993). Ecological models of human development. In M. Gauvain & M. Cole (Eds.), *Readings on the development of children* (2nd ed., Freeman. (Reprinted from International Encyclopedia of Education, Vol. 3, 2nd Ed, 1994, pp. 37–43). Elsevier.

Centers for Disease Control and Prevention. (2013). CDC health disparities and inequalities report—United States, 2013. *Morbidity and Mortality Weekly Report*, *62*(3), 1–187. https://www.cdc.gov/mmwr/pdf/other/su6203.pdf

Centers for Disease Control and Prevention. (2020, April 15). *Coronavirus disease 2019 (COVID-19).* https://www.cdc.gov/coronavirus/2019-ncov/need-extra-precautions/people-at-higher-risk.html

Choi, E., Ospina, J., Steger, M. F., & Orsi, R. (2018). Understanding work enjoyment among older workers: The significance of flexible work options and age discrimination in the workplace. *Journal of Gerontological Social Work*, *61*(8), 867–886. https://doi.org/10.1080/01634372.2018.1515140

Choi, E., Tang, F., & Copeland, V. C. (2017). Racial/ethnic inequality among older workers: Focusing on whites, blacks, and Latinos within the cumulative advantage/disadvantage framework. *Journal of Social Service Research*, *43*(1), 18–36. https://doi.org/10.1080/01488376.2016.1235068

Cohn, D., & Passel, J. S. (2018). *A record 64 million Americans live in multigenerational households.* Pew Research Center. https://www.pewresearch.org/fact-tank/2018/04/05/a-record-64-million-americans-live in multigenerational-households/

Crystal, S., Shea, D. G., & Reyes, A. M. (2017). Cumulative advantage, cumulative disadvantage, and evolving patterns of late-life inequality. *The Gerontologist*, *57*(5), 910–920. https://doi.org/10.1093/geront/gnw056

Davis, M. T., Warfield, M. E., Boguslaw, J., Roundtree-Swain, D., & Kellogg, G. (2020). Parenting a 6 year old is not what I planned in retirement: Trauma and stress among grandparents due to the opioid crisis. *Journal of Gerontological Social Work.* Advance online publication. https://doi.org/10.1080/01634372.2020.1752872

Dingemans, E., Henkens, K., & Van Solinge, H. (2016). Access to bridge employment: Who finds and who does not find work after retirement? *The Gerontologist, 56*(4), 630–640. https://doi.org/10.1093/geront/gnu182

Fortuna, K. L., Torous, J., Depp, C. A., Jimenez, D. E., Areán, P. A., Walker, R., Ajilore, O., Goldstein, C. M., Cosco, T. D., Brooks, J. M., Vahia, I. V., & Bartels, S. J. (2019). A future research agenda for digital geriatric mental healthcare. *The American Journal of Geriatric Psychiatry, 27*(11), 1277–1285. https://doi.org/10.1016/j.jagp.2019.05.013

Gonzales, E., Lee, K., & Harootyan, B. (2020). Voices from the field: Ecological factors that promote employment and health among low-income older adults with implications for direct social work practice. *Clinical Social Work Journal, 48*(2), 211–222. https://doi.org/10.1007/s10615-019-00719-x

Gould, E. (2020, March 31). *Older workers can't work from home and are at a higher risk for COVID-19. Economic Policy Institute.* https://www.epi.org/blog/older-workers-cant-work-from-home-and-at-high-risk-for-covid-19/

Halvorsen, C. J. (2019). *What does it mean to have a society with more older people than younger ones?* Encore.org, Boston College School of Social Work, and Center on Aging & Work at Boston College. https://encore.org/halvorsen-report/

Halvorsen, C. J., & Chen, Y.-C. (2019). The diversity of interest in later-life entrepreneurship: Results from a nationally representative survey of Americans aged 50 to 70. *PloS One, 14*(6), e0217971. https://doi.org/10.1371/journal.pone.0217971

Halvorsen, C. J., & Emerman, J. (2014). The encore movement: Baby boomers and older adults building community. *Generations, 37*(4), 33–39. https://www.asaging.org/blog/encore-movement-baby-boomers-and-older-adults-can-be-powerful-force-build-community

Halvorsen, C. J., & Morrow-Howell, N. (2017). A conceptual framework on self-employment in later life: Toward a research agenda. *Work, Aging and Retirement, 3*(4), 313–324. https://doi.org/10.1093/workar/waw031

Halvorsen, C. J., & Skees, S. (2019). Financial capability in later life. In S. Sanders, S. R. Kolomer, C. Waites Spellman, & V. M. Rizzo (Eds.), *Gerontological social work and the grand challenges* (pp. 157–168). Springer International Publishing. https://doi.org/10.1007/978-3-030-26334-8_11

Halvorsen, C. J., & Yulikova, O. (2020). Job training and so much more for low-income older adults: The senior community service employment program. *Clinical Social Work Journal, 48*(2), 223–229. https://doi.org/10.1007/s10615-019-00734-y

Health Equity Works. (2014). *Videos.* Brown School at Washington University in St. Louis. https://healthequityworks.wustl.edu/publications/videos/

Johnson, R. (2012). *Older workers, retirement, and the Great Recession.* Stanford Center on Poverty and Inequality. https://web.stanford.edu/group/recessiontrends/cgi-bin/web/sites/all/themes/barron/pdf/Retirement_fact_sheet.pdf

Johnson, R., & Gosselin, P. (2018). *How secure is employment at older ages?* (Research report). Urban Institute. https://www.urban.org/sites/default/files/publication/99570/how_secure_is_employment_at_older_ages_2.pdf

Kondrat, M. E. (2002). Actor-centered social work: Re-visioning "person-in-environment" through a critical theory lens. *Social Work, 47*(4), 435–448. https://doi.org/10.1093/sw/47.4.435

Lubben, J., Gironda, M., Sabbath, E., Kong, J., & Johnson, C. (2015). *Social isolation presents a grand challenges for social work* (Working Paper No. 7; Grand Challenges for Social Work Initiative. American Academy of Social Work and Social Welfare). https://grandchallengesforsocialwork.org/wp-content/uploads/2015/12/WP8-with-cover.pdf

Massachusetts Executive Office of Health and Human Services. (2020). *Learn about the community tracing collaborative*. Mass.Gov. https://www.mass.gov/info-details/learn-about-the-community-tracing-collaborative

Mikelson, K. S. (2017). *The role of SCSEP in workforce training for low-income older workers* (White paper). Urban Institute. https://www.urban.org/sites/default/files/publication/94371/2001575_scsep_white_paper_finalized_2.pdf

Morrow-Howell, N. (2010). Volunteering in later life: Research frontiers. *The Journals of Gerontology. Series B, Psychological Sciences and Social Sciences, 65B*(4), 461–469. https://doi.org/10.1093/geronb/gbq024

Morrow-Howell, N., Halvorsen, C. J., Hovmand, P., Lee, C., & Ballard, E. (2017). Conceptualizing productive engagement in a system dynamics perspective. *Innovation in Aging, 1*(1), igx018. https://doi.org/10.1093/geroni/igx018

Morrow-Howell, N., Galucia, N., & Swinford, E. (2020). Recovering from the COVID-19 pandemic: A focus on older adults. *Journal of Aging & Social Policy*. Advance online publication. https://doi.org/10.1080/08959420.2020.1759758

Morrow-Howell, N., Gonzales, E., Matz-Costa, C., & Greenfield, E. A. (2015). *Increasing productive engagement in later life* (Working Paper No. 8; Grand Challenges for Social Work Initiative). American Academy of Social Work and Social Welfare. https://grandchallengesforsocialwork.org/wp-content/uploads/2015/12/WP8-with-cover.pdf

National Center for Health Statistics. (2018). *Health, United States, 2017: With special feature on mortality*. U.S. Department of Health and Human Services. https://www.cdc.gov/nchs/data/hus/hus17.pdf

Perrin, A., & Turner, E. (2019). *Smartphones help blacks, Hispanics bridge some – But not all – Digital gaps with whites*. Pew Research Center. https://www.pewresearch.org/fact-tank/2019/08/20/smartphones-help-blacks-hispanics-bridge-some-but-not-all-digital-gaps-with-whites/

Pitt-Catsouphes, M., McNamara, T. K., James, J., & Halvorsen, C. J. (2017). Innovative pathways to meaningful work: Older adults as volunteers and self-employed entrepreneurs. In J. McCarthy & E. Parry (Eds.), *The Palgrave handbook of age diversity and work* (pp. 195–224). Palgrave Macmillan.

Sliva, S. M., Greenfield, J. C., Bender, K., & Freedenthal, S. (2019). Introduction to the special section on public impact scholarship in social work: A conceptual review and call to action. *Journal of the Society for Social Work and Research, 10*(4), 529–544. https://doi.org/10.1086/706112

Swinford, E., Galucia, N., & Morrow-Howell, N. (2020). Applying gerontological social work perspectives to the coronavirus pandemic. *Journal of Gerontological Social Work*. Advance online publication. https://doi.org/10.1080/01634372.2020.1766628

Tankersley, J., & Savage, C. (2020, April 28). Businesses seek sweeping shield from pandemic liability before they reopen. *The New York Times*. https://www.nytimes.com/2020/04/28/business/businesses-coronavirus-liability.html

U.S. Centers for Medicare & Medicaid Services. (2020). *Medicare & coronavirus*. Medicare.Gov. https://www.medicare.gov/medicare-coronavirus

U.S. Department of Health & Human Services. (2014, September 11). *Who is eligible for medicare?* HHS.Gov. https://www.hhs.gov/answers/medicare-and-medicaid/who-is-elibible-for-medicare/index.html

U.S. Department of Labor, Employment & Training Administration. (2018a). *PY 2017 participant evaluation of SCSEP*. https://www.doleta.gov/Seniors/pdf/Participant_Survey_Report/PY2017_Nationwide_Participant_Survey_Report.pdf

U.S. Department of Labor, Employment & Training Administration. (2018b, August 20). *Senior community service employment program*. https://www.doleta.gov/seniors/

U.S. Department of Labor, Employment & Training Administration. (2018c). *Nationwide quarterly progress report: PY 2018.* https://www.doleta.gov/Seniors/html_docs/Docs/PY%2018%20QPR%20final.pdf

U.S. Department of Labor, Employment & Training Administration. (2019). *Senior community service employment program analysis of service to minority individuals, PY 2017 [Vol. I].* https://www.dol.gov/sites/dolgov/files/ETA/Seniors/pdfs/PY_2017_SCSEP_Minority_Report_Vol_I.pdf

U.S. Department of Labor, Employment & Training Administration. (2020). *ETA coronavirus (COVID-19) FAQs: Senior Community Service Employment Program (SCSEP).* WorkforceGPS. https://www.workforcegps.org/-/media/Global-Site/Content/Resources/COVID-FAQs/SCSEP_FAQs_COVID_19_20200429.ashx

Vogels, E. A. (2019). *Millennials stand out for their technology use, but older generations also embrace digital life.* Pew Research Center. https://www.pewresearch.org/fact-tank/2019/09/09/us-generations-technology-use/

Yancura, L. A. (2013). Service use and unmet service needs in grandparents raising grandchildren. *Journal of Gerontological Social Work, 56*(6), 473–486. https://doi.org/10.1080/01634372.2013.804471

Zendell, A. L., Fortune, A. E., Mertz, L. K. P., & Koelewyn, N. (2007). University-community partnerships in gerontological social work: Building consensus around student learning. *Journal of Gerontological Social Work, 50*(1–2), 155–172. https://doi.org/10.1300/J083v50n01_11

Caregiving in Times of Uncertainty: Helping Adult Children of Aging Parents Find Support during the COVID-19 Outbreak

Elizabeth Lightfoot ⓘ and Rajean P. Moone

ABSTRACT

The COVID-19 pandemic, which is especially dangerous to older people, has disrupted the lives of older people and their family caregivers. This commentary outlines the adaptive and emerging practices in formal supportive services for family caregivers, the changing types of support that family caregivers are providing to their older relatives, and the ways family caregivers are seeking informal caregiving support during the COVID-19 outbreak.

COVID-19, first diagnosed in Wuhan Province in China in 2019, is especially dangerous to older people because of age-related health conditions and age-related declines in their immune systems. Early studies put the mortality rate of COVID-19 for people between ages 70 and 79 years at 8%, and for those over age 80 at 14.8% (Wu & McGoogan, 2020). In the United States, The Centers for Disease Control and Prevention (CDC) (Centers for Disease Control, 2020) estimates that eight out of ten deaths have been among people ages 65 and older. Older adults living in long-term care facilities, such as nursing homes or assisted living facilities, are at a very high risk for mortality from COVID-19, particularly with asymptomatic or presymptomatic workers inadvertently spreading the virus in the facilities (McMichael et al., 2020). While national data were unavailable as of early May 2020, seven states reported more than half of their COVID-19 deaths were residents of long-term care facilities (Kaiser Family Foundation, 2020), with some states reporting much higher rates, such as in Minnesota where about 80% of its deaths were from long-term care facilities (Minnesota Department of Health, 2020).

In response to older people's higher chances of complications from COVID-19, the CDC (Centers for Disease Control, 2020) has recommended older people living in community settings to stay home as much as possible, and when venturing outside, to practice "social distancing." The CDC's (Centers for Disease Control, 2020) guidance to long-term care facilities urged facilities to restrict visitors unless visiting a dying relative, screen workers and residents for symptoms, require workers to wear cloth masks, and limit activities for residents. When long-term care facilities have COVID-19 within their facility, they are advised to separate those with and without COVID-19 through quarantines and cohorting, which often results in residents being mostly confined to their rooms. While all of this is challenging for older people living in the community and long-term facilities, it also can create enormous stress and challenges for their caregivers. This commentary outlines adaptive and emerging practices in formal supportive services for caregivers, the changing types of support that family caregivers are providing to their older relatives, and the ways family caregivers are seeking informal caregiving support during this global pandemic. Information was obtained from professional and personal experience, feedback from interactions with over 670 caregivers through a series of webinars co-presented by the authors at university and nonprofit venues, and discussions with caregivers in several online elder caregiving support groups hosted by the authors.

Family caregiving

An estimated 41 million family caregivers[1] provide 34 billion hours of care to other adults in the United States. This care is valued at over 470 USD billion annually (AARP Public Policy Institute, 2019). Caregiving touches nearly all Americans in some way. Rosalyn Carter is famously quoted as saying, "There are only four kinds of people in the world. Those who have been caregivers. Those who are currently caregivers. Those who will be caregivers, and those who will need a caregiver (Snelling, 2012)." The care provided informally by family can take many forms, such as providing assistance with activities of daily living or offering social and emotional support. The care can occur in a variety of settings, including a care receiver's home, the caregiver's home, an assisted living establishment, or a nursing home. Family caregivers provide, on average, 20 hours per week of care for a period of nearly 5 years, with roughly one-third providing care to more than one older person living in the community (Gaugler & Kane, 2015). Trends in family caregiving of older people living in the community show declines as the population ages and successive generations have less children (Stone, 2015), which can put more responsibility on a smaller number of caregivers, as well as an increased

---

[1]The authors recognize that there are numerous ways to define "caregivers." For the purposes of this article, "family caregivers" are defined as friends and families that provide care to an older adult. They may receive some compensation for this care (such as a consumer directed plan), but it is generally not considered a career. This is in contrast to paid direct care workers who can often be referred to as formal or paid "caregivers."

reliance on formal systems to provide care. With COVID-19, family caregivers of older adults in community settings are often providing this care from a distance.

Family members also provide care to older relatives living who are living in long-term care settings, including nursing homes and assisted living facilities. These caregivers spend about as much time with their relatives as do those caring for those in community settings (Port et al., 2005). As there are significant staffing shortages in long-term care settings (Geng et al., 2019), which have been exacerbated by COVID-19 (Mettler et al., 2020), family caregivers of those living in formal settings might feel extra stress worrying about the care their family member is receiving and a sense of helplessness at their lack of ability to monitor their care.

Supportive services for caregivers during COVID-19

Crucial to successful caregiving is the utilization of supportive services designed to decrease burden, stress, depression and burnout (Iecovich, 2008). While studies about caregiving and COVID-19 are not yet available, it is highly likely that due to a combination of social distancing, shelter-in-place or stay-at-home orders,[2] and the disproportionate impact of the virus on older adults, caregivers of adults living both in community and long-term care are in need of different types of formal caregiving supports. The following details the emerging changes to formal supportive services during the COVID-19 crisis.

The 2000 Older Americans Act reauthorization included a provision to support informal caregivers known as the National Family Caregiver Support Program (Title III-E). The passage of Title III-E acknowledged the crucial role caregivers play in the lives of older Americans. Funding through the Older Americans Act flows to states and area agencies on aging, who then develop relationships with providers in the community to offer direct support to caregivers.

Eligibility for Title III-E mirrors most of the Older Americans Act Titles with some uniqueness. Services are available to people 18 years and older providing care to someone 60 years and older or someone of any age with dementia. The program also supports relative caregivers 55 years and older who are providing care to children or adults with disabilities (Administration for Community Living, 2019). Also similar to the other Titles, a Title III-E provider cannot charge for services, but can request either a voluntary contribution or utilize a quasi-sliding fee scale known as cost-sharing. Services cannot be denied due to a caregiver's inability or unwillingness to pay. The

---

[2]The majority of states and many cities in the United States implemented a variety of temporary orders requiring or requesting residents to stay-at-home or shelter-in-place. There was no uniformity to the language used to described these orders, and great variability in their length and coverage (Mervosh et al. (2020).

CARES (Coronavirus Aid, Relieve and Economic Security) Act included an additional 100 USD million for Title III-E (Administration for Community Living, 2020).

Services available under Title III-E are comprehensive and include coaching and counseling, support groups, education, respite care, adult day services, and supplemental services. Supplemental services are services that often target the care receiver, but benefit the caregiver in some way. For example, a care receiver may need their lawn mowed and the primary caregiver may not be able to provide this service, but it is crucial in order for the caregiver to continue to provide care. Another agency could be engaged to offer the lawn mowing service as a way to support the caregiver so they can continue to provide other care.

The response to COVID-19 has greatly affected the delivery of formal systems and supports for caregivers. For example, one crucial support for caregivers is adult day services, where an older adult attends a day program that provides socialization and health related services. Adult day services provide critical respite for caregivers who may be employed or have a number of other tasks that need to be accomplished (such as grocery shopping, medical appointments, caring for young children, etc.). In many states adult day services have been closed due to stay-at-home orders, such as in Minnesota, where all 225 adult day service programs were closed, displacing thousands of older adults, many of whom experience cognitive and memory impairment, who attended adult day programs during the week. Service providers have needed to innovate quickly and continue to practice nimble, flexible project management to continue to support caregivers. The following is a case example of how one service provider has adapted its services to provide caregiving support.

FamilyMeans

Adaptation and innovation in service delivery

FamilyMeans is a nonprofit social services agency in Washington County in Minnesota. As a recipient of an Older Americans Act Title III-E contract, the organization provides a comprehensive array of services and supports for caregivers. During the COVID-19 crisis and stay-at-home orders, FamilyMeans caregiver support staff have begun to initiate a number of telesupport services including:

- Conducting caregiver consultation over phone, Skype or Zoom. Anecdotally, themes of increased stress due to stay-at-home orders, lack of in-person respite, and facility visiting restrictions have begun to emerge.

- Contacting individual clients via phone and writing notes to ensure needs are being met and connections continue.
- Providing in-home respite through volunteers over telephone and video-conference. One volunteer found a streaming movie that a particular care receiver would enjoy. They watched it simultaneously while the caregiver had a break for a couple of hours.
- Offering online videos with messages from staff for respite care participants. The videos are 20 minutes long and offer some social interaction and familiar faces for people with memory loss.
- Holding Memory Cafes via zoom. Memory Cafes are lunches supported by local restaurants for people living with dementia and their caregivers. With restaurants closed, these Cafes have moved to a virtual setting.
- Holding Zoom coffee breaks with staff where anyone can join for drop-in support.
- Increasing e-mail communication to weekly posts which include ideas for activities that can be done from home (such as exploring a live eagle cam, online exercise classes, and a self-care resource developed by mental health staff).

Services funded by Title III-E may differ in availability and response to COVID-19 and connecting caregivers to local supports is necessary. Finding a caregiver support provider is a phone call or mouse click away. Nationally caregivers can contact the Eldercare Locator which can connect them to local information and assistance programs offered through states and area agencies on aging.

Informal caregiving supports during COVID-19

Caregivers of older people living in community and long-term care settings are also changing the types of support that they provide to older relatives as well as the ways that they are seeking informal support for themselves in response to COVID-19. The following details some of the emerging types of informal care that caregivers are providing from a distance, ways caregivers are seeking their own support, and examples of caregiver individual and systems advocacy to bring awareness to the impact of COVID-19 on senior care communities.

Providing informal caregiving from a distance

Staying connected

Caregivers have quickly adopted new ways of connecting with older relatives, often supported with new technology. While family caregivers already used telephone and/or video calls to connect with their older relatives, often to supplement in-person visits, this now has become the main way many caregivers are staying connected with their relatives in community or long-term care settings. Video calls have become especially popular, with care-givers using these calls to substitute for in-person visits, as well as a means to reduce the social isolation of older people who are not able to participate in their typical social activities. Older residents might have their own tablets, such as an iPad, use a specially designed tablet geared toward older people, such as *GrandPads*, or use facility owned tablets. For those living in facilities, workers can help residents establish connections with these devices. Caregivers can also use these, or other devices, such as laptops, for playing interactive games together, listening to concerts or shows together, or doing other online activities together. Some caregivers and older relatives are not as comfortable with smart phones or tablets, or are not able to afford this type of technology, and instead rely on traditional phone calls. Caregivers are making use of lower-technology too, such as letter writing or setting up penpals with family members, friends or grandchildren. There are also a variety of new ways to connect in-person, while maintaining social distan-cing. For example, some long-term care facilities are arranging window-greetings, where caregivers stand outside the window and either wave or talk on the phone with their older caregivers, and family members are visiting their older relatives through various forms of distant visits (driving their cars by the facility while honking, singing to residents who are standing on a balcony, etc.)

Arranging delivery of essential items

Family caregivers have also taken on the responsibilities of arranging for delivery of essential items, such as food or medication. For those caring for residents living in the community, this activity keeps their older relatives from having to shop or otherwise venture in the community. Family members might be doing the errands themselves, or arranging for a delivery service to send needed items. Family caregivers caring for those in long-term care settings also are delivering essential items, including items that the long-term care facility is no longer able to procure during the pandemic.

Providing activities and information

Caregivers are also providing activities to loved ones that can help reduce social isolation and fill the void left by the cancellation of their typical activities. The types of activities are personalized based on their loved one's interests and cognitive ability. Examples include books, puzzles, craft materials, and devices for watching movies or shows or listening to audio books. For those with more significant cognitive decline, activities could include a portable music player with a playlist of their loved one's favorite songs, photobooks or videos of family or friends, or fidget blankets. Caregivers are also providing information to their older relatives about COVID-19, such as the latest news on transmission, prevention and treatment, or state and local ordinances, particularly for those who are not able to access news and information online.

Thanking long-term care workers

As caregivers are no longer able to visit long-term care settings during the Covid-19 crisis, the workers in these facilities are having to take on an additional supportive role. Workers, who are often risking their own health to provide care for residents in long-term care settings, have become the main source of social interaction for residents, particularly in facilities where residents have been quarantined in their rooms. Caregivers are providing support for these workers in a variety of ways, such as sending thank you notes or small gifts.

Monitoring from afar

One key activity that family caregivers typically do for older relatives in long-term care facilities is to monitor the quality of care they are receiving. Caregivers are having to find new ways to monitor when they are not able to visit, such as through increased communication with workers and their supervisors, or monitoring while connecting with their loved one through video or phone chats.

Taking action

Some family caregivers have been involved in advocacy efforts related to protecting loved ones during the COVID-19 outbreak as well as protecting and supporting their paid caregivers. This advocacy has been at multiple levels, including advocating at the institutional level for long-term care facilities to adopt procedures to protect residents, such as requiring all workers in a nursing home to wear masks or increasing transparency about the number of residents who have tested positive for COVID-19; or at the state level, such as demanding that states include protections for residents of long-term care facilities or provide COVID-19 testing at all facilities throughout the state. Family caregivers have become community organizing and advocacy leaders for protecting older people during COVID-19. Community advocacy activities have included petitioning stores to have special hours or to require masks, organizing mask drives to provide personal protective equipment for senior care workers, or leading parades and concerts outside senior communities. Other caregivers have taken their voices to the media, contacting reporters to publicize the COVID-19 outbreaks in long-term care facilities and pointing out the lack of a swift government response. They have shared both positive and negative experiences in news articles and blogs. All of these can lead to policy changes and help build community and support during uncertain times.

Getting informal caregiving support during COVID-19

While formal aging services programs are adapting to provide formal support for caregivers during the COVID-19 outbreak, caregivers are also finding new ways to get informal support for themselves. Many caregivers rely only on informal supports for their caregiving, while others rely on a combination on formal and informal supports to assist them in caregiving (Chow et al., 2010). The following describes key ways family members are seeking informal supports.

Coordinating with other family members and friends

Caregivers of older adults have always had to coordinate and negotiate caregiving responsibilities with other family members and friends, and other families and friends are often the main source of caregiving support. During COVID-19, the focus of this coordination and support has changed. Caregivers are now having to coordinate care from a distance, such as scheduling regular communication through phone or video to help reduce social isolation. This can also involve having families and friends making important decisions regarding whether to remove their family members from a long-term care facility because of the dangers of COVID-19, often with very incomplete information. Some extended families are developing COVID-19 plans to assist them in providing care and making decisions from a distance.

Online informal support

As in-person support groups are not available, many formal services have developed telephone or video support groups for caregivers. Another type of informal, peer-led support group has emerged: support groups on social media platforms. These support groups, which are not facilitated by service providers or long-term care facilities, can give caregivers a more open forum to not only provide each support, but to assist caregivers who might be frustrated with facilities or service providers. Using social media for social support is particular relevant for caregivers who are seeking caregiving support for the first time during stay-at-home orders, as this type of support is available in real-time, and also can lead to a sense of empowerment among participants who can share and access resources through these venues (Ammari & Schoenebeck, 2015). The informal COVID-19 era caregiving support groups on social media have also fostered advocacy on behalf of older family members. This type of support, while useful, is only accessible to those who have the appropriate technology.

Recognizing competing responsibilities

Caregivers are also recognizing the competing sources of stress during the COVID-19 crisis. Not only are they worried about providing care from a distance to their older relatives, they are also worried about the health of their family members who are at a high risk of death if they become infected with COVID-19 because of their age and/or age-related health conditions. For those whose loved ones are living in long-term care facilities, there is the compounded stress of the high rates of COVID-19 within such facilities. With the required social distancing, family caregivers can have a heightened sense of helplessness because they are not able to protect their family members or provide the type or amount of care that they want to provide. In addition, caregivers might simultaneously be adjusting to working at home, caring for children who are home from school, coping with losing their job or some of their income due to state or city stay-at-home rules or the economic downturn, and/or experiencing serious financial problems. Caregivers also worry about becoming infected with COVID-19 themselves, or about other family members and friends. All of these stressors make caregiving for older family members during this global pandemic difficult.

Conclusion

There is much we do not know about the course of this pandemic and the long term impacts on our communities, and gerontological research efforts on the effects of COVID-19 on caregiving are just beginning. We know that COVID-19 will continue to transform the delivery of long-term services and supports, including caregiver support, as well as the ways we interact with our loved ones into the future. For older adults and their caregivers, social distancing and fear may also continue when many have returned to work and the social distancing restrictions are lifted. Gerontological research is needed to examine which types of formal caregiving supports are needed and most effective during crises such as COVID-19, and which emerging caregiving supports should be retained after this crisis ends. The field of social work must be particularly attuned and sensitive to the needs of family caregivers who may be experiencing added burden, stress, and depression, and the differences in needs based on a variety family circumstances. Connecting caregivers to formal supports like the Title III-E network, as well as offering suggestions for continued connection with their family members and for finding informal sources of support, is helpful both during the global pandemic and after.

ORCID

Elizabeth Lightfoot ⓘ http://orcid.org/0000-0002-0861-1047

References

AARP Public Policy Institute. (2019, November). *Valuing the invaluable 2019 Update: Charting a path forward.* Washington: AARP Public Policy Institute. https://www.aarp. org/content/dam/aarp/ppi/2019/11/understanding-the-contributions-of-family-caregivers-infographic.doi.10.26419-2Fppi.00082.003.pdf

Administration for Community Living. (2019). *National family caregiver support program.* Washington: Administration for Community Living. https://acl.gov/programs/support-caregivers/national-family-caregiver-support-program

Administration for Community Living. (2020, March 29). *Supporting community living during COVID-19: CARES act and civil rights protections.* Washington: Administration for Community Living. https://acl.gov/news-and-events/announcements/supporting-community-living-during-covid-19-cares-act-and-civil

Ammari, T., & Schoenebeck, S. (2015, April). Networked empowerment on Facebook groups for parents of children with special needs. In *Proceedings of the 33rd annual ACM conference on human factors in computing systems* . Seoul, South Korea. (pp. 2805–2814).

Centers for Disease Control. (2020, April). *Older adults: Coronavirus disease 2019 (COVID-19).* Atlanta: Centers for Disease Control. https://www.cdc.gov/coronavirus/2019-ncov/need-extra-precautions/older-adults.html

Chow, J. C. C., Auh, E. Y., Scharlach, A. E., Lehning, A. J., & Goldstein, C. (2010). Types and sources of support received by family caregivers of older adults from diverse racial and ethnic groups. *Journal of Ethnic & Cultural Diversity in Social Work, 19*(3), 175–194. https://doi.org/10.1080/15313204.2010.499318

Gaugler, J. E., & Kane, R. L. (Eds.). (2015). *Family caregiving in the new normal.* Academic Press.

Geng, F., Stevenson, D. G., & Grabowski, D. C. (2019). Daily nursing home staffing levels highly variable, often below CMS expectations. *Health Affairs, 38*(7), 1095–1100. https://doi.org/10.1377/hlthaff.2018.05322

Iecovich, E. (2008). Caregiving burden, community services, and quality of life of primary caregivers of frail elderly persons. *Journal of Applied Gerontology, 27*(3), 309–330. https://doi.org/10.1177/0733464808315289

Kaiser Family Foundation. (2020, May 2). *COVID-19: Confirmed cases and deaths by state.* Washington: Kaiser Family Foundation. https://www.kff.org/health-costs/issue-brief/state-data-and-policy-actions-to-address-coronavirus/

McMichael, T. M., Currie, D. W., Clark, S., Pogosjans, S., Kay, M., Schwartz, N. G., … Ferro, J. (2020). Epidemiology of covid-19 in a long-term care facility in King County, Washington. *New England Journal of Medicine.* https://doi.org/10.1056/NEJMoa2005412

Mervosh, S., Lu, D., & Swales, V. (2020, April 20). See which states and cities have told residents to stay at home. *New York Times.* https://www.nytimes.com/interactive/2020/us/coronavirus-stay-at-home-order.html

Mettler, K., Hernandez, A. R., Wan, W., & Bernstein, L. (2020, March 5). Health care workers worry about coronavirus protection. *The Washington Post.* https://www.washingtonpost.

com/health/health-care-workers-worry-about-coronavirus-protection/2020/03/05/
be04d5a8-5e33-11ea-9055-5fa12981bbbf_story.html

Minnesota Department of Health. (2020, May 2). *Situation update for coronavirus disease 2019 (COVID-19)*. St. Paul: Minnesota Department of Health. https://www.health.state.mn. us/diseases/coronavirus/situation.html

Port, C. L., Zimmerman, S., Williams, C. S., Dobbs, D., Preisser, J. S., & Williams, S. W. (2005). Families filling the gap: Comparing family involvement for assisted living and nursing home residents with dementia. *The Gerontologist, 45*(suppl_1), 87–95. https://doi. org/10.1093/geront/45.suppl_1.87

Snelling, S. (2012, August 6). *Rosalyn carter: A pioneering caregiving advocate says more must be done*. Next Avenue. https://www.nextavenue.org/rosalynn-carter-pioneering-caregiving-advocate-says-more-must-be-done/

Stone, R. I. (2015). Factors affecting the future of family caregiving in the United States. In Gaugler, J. E., & Kane, R. L. (Eds.). *Family caregiving in the new normal* (pp. 57–77). Academic Press.

Wu, Z., & McGoogan, J. M. (2020). Characteristics of and important lessons from the coronavirus disease 2019 (COVID-19) outbreak in China: Summary of a report of 72 314 cases from the Chinese center for disease control and prevention. *JAMA, 323*(13), 1239–1242. https://doi.org/10.1001/jama.2020.2648

Part II

Gerontological Social Work Role in Addressing COVID-19

Gerontological Social Work's Pivotal Role in the COVID-19 Pandemic: A Response from AGESW Leadership

Dear Editor,

The COVID-19 pandemic is putting a spotlight on older adults, a population that many social workers, ourselves included, devote entire careers to. Whether in research, teaching, or community programming, older adults, including our family members and friends and possibly ourselves, face an increased risk at this time (Centers for Disease Control and Prevention, 2020). Despite this increased risk, older people, just like people of any age, want to remain active and engaged in their families, communities, and paid work.

National social work organizations are highlighting ways to support populations particularly vulnerable to this coronavirus pandemic. Both the National Association of Social Workers (2020) and the Council on Social Work Education (2020) offer information about supporting clients – particularly older adults – as well as supporting the agencies that deliver services, social work professionals, and students. Policy and practice matters are at the heart of social work. Promoting equitable and expanded access to testing, advocating for paid leave for those who are self-isolating or sick, and standing against marginalization because of age, gender, race, ethnicity, sexual orientation, gender identity, disability status, and citizenship, among others, are all social justice concerns related to this pandemic.

Now, more than ever, gerontological social workers can use their voices and actions to reduce the ageism that so many older adults are facing and to advocate for older people being viewed and discussed with dignity. We must move beyond the counting of cases and deaths to acknowledging the lived experiences of everyone affected by COVID-19. At the local, regional, and national levels, there continue to be urgent opportunities to advocate for timely and accurate information dissemination to older adults and their caregivers.

Many of the inequities we are seeing through this pandemic have long been present in our communities, institutions, and society. They are often complex problems resulting from systemic bias and discrimination, including ageism and racism and their intersectionality, that are present at the micro, mezzo, and macro levels. Indeed, the NASW Code of Ethics (National Association of Social Workers, 2018) states that "fundamental to social work is attention to the environmental forces that create, contribute to, and address problems in living" (preamble para. 1).

These forces can increase the risks of exposure to and complications from COVID-19. Racism at the individual and institutional levels compounds these risks, creating a system that leads to higher rates of unjustified uses of force and violence against Black people in the United States (Ehrenfeld & Harris, 2020), higher rates of incarceration for people of color (Gramlich, 2020), and higher rates of COVID-19 among those incarcerated (Akiyama et al., 2020), highlighting the public health risks of racism. The COVID-19 pandemic, with its devastating effect on older adults and people of color in the U.S., has shed great light on how inequity has led to extreme differences in illness and mortality rates (National Center for Health Statistics, 2020; Swinford et al., 2020).

Grand challenges for social work

AGESW members, their colleagues, and students have been active in numerous ways during this crisis in various cities. Many have submitted letters and commentaries to the *Journal of Gerontological Social Work* and many more are working to address the Grand Challenges for Social Work, including the newest Grand Challenge to Eliminate Racism, announced in June 2020 (Grand Challenges for Social Work, 2020). We recently issued a call to our members to alert us to their responses to addressing the challenges of COVID-19. While only a snapshot into the work of our members, we include some examples below, with their corresponding Grand Challenge for Social Work, which we believe will inspire those working to enhance the well-being of older adults in the U.S. and around the globe.

Grand challenge: close the health gap

Of the 48 Geriatric Workforce Enhancement Programs (GWEPs) in the country, only three teams have social workers in leading roles. Marla Berg-Weger (St. Louis University), Scott Wilks (Louisiana State University), and Keith Anderson (University of Montana) are all involved in providing telehealth programs such as dementia caregiver support groups and education and training for interdisciplinary professionals and students on COVID-19. Holly Dabelko-Schoeny and colleagues (The Ohio State University) are working to address food insecurity, loneliness, and household necessities through its Age-Friendly Columbus and Franklin County initiative, which is also offering a Friendly Phone Line for older adults to call. AGESW past president, Sara Sanders (University of Iowa), is facilitating weekly state-wide meetings for nursing home social workers in Iowa.

Grand challenges: eradicate social isolation and harness technology for social good

New York City was devastated in the early months of COVID-19. Created in response to the shelter in place orders at the beginning of March 2020, Ernest Gonzales and Stacey Gordon (New York University) are working with the intergenerational Neighbor to Neighbor Volunteer Corps that engages younger and older residents in faculty housing. Volunteers make weekly check-in telephone calls to their neighbors, share food and healthcare resources, and offer to connect their neighbors to an NYU Silver School of Social Work faculty member or doctoral student for mental wellness check-ins. This initiative is also collaborating with CyberSeniors, an organization that provides meaningful intergenerational interaction through mentorship between students and older adults who teach each other technology and life skills. In another city hard hit by the pandemic, AGESW president, Tam Perry (Wayne State University) worked with colleagues to create a telephone outreach program to reach 1,300 seniors in the city (Rorai & Perry, 2020). A social work graduate student at the University of Georgia, Kim Wolf, created a website of COVID activities for homebound older adults (www.engagemen tactivities.com). She also recognized, through her own personal experience, the isolation that nursing home residents were experiencing and created a virtual pet visit program for residents in congregate living (https://news. uga.edu/grad-student-pets-together-group-homes/).

Grand challenge: build financial capability for all

AGESW board member Cal Halvorsen (Boston College) is collaborating with leadership of the Massachusetts Senior Community Service Employment Program (SCSEP), the only federal workforce training program designed for older workers, to understand the role of SCSEP in the well-being of participants and how the COVID-19 pandemic has affected low-income older adults seeking paid work (Halvorsen & Yulikova, 2020a, 2020b). A virtual participatory research project will take place this summer.

Grand challenge: create social responses to a changing environment

Social workers often take on the fundamental challenge of direct service and macro practice for the same communities simultaneously. Mercedes Bern-

Klug (University of Iowa) and members of the National Nursing Home Social Work Research Group, including AGESW vice president Nancy Kusmaul (University of Maryland Baltimore County) and additional gerontological social work faculty, started meeting weekly to discuss how to help nursing home social workers in practice. They cultivated resources and provided online support sessions (Kusmaul et al., 2020). Tam Perry discussed her work with a multidisciplinary coalition to assess and build capacity to meet the needs of people living in low-income senior housing in the Detroit, both for current needs related to COVID-19 and the projected second wave of the pandemic (Archambault et al., in press).

In these unprecedented times, AGESW members have been responsive to the population we serve. AGESW provides leadership in the areas of gerontological social work education, research, and policy, while fostering cooperation, collegiality, and an exchange of ideas among social work educators, researchers, and students committed to or interested in gerontology (Association for Gerontology Education in Social Work, 2020). In response to the COVID-19 pandemic, AGESW as an organization has established programming to meet the needs of its members, such as virtual town halls and webinars on nursing home social work and COVID-19 and addressing loneliness and social isolation among older adults during the COVID-19 pandemic. AGESW is also providing virtual mentoring space for doctoral students with a focus on gerontology to support their academic work during these challenging times, including a recent webinar on how to publish within the *Journal of Gerontological Social Work*, available on AGESW's website.

We invite others to engage with the work of AGESW to build our shared capacity, care skillfully, and teach empathetically to meet another important Grand Challenge for Social Work: to Advance Long and Productive Lives.

Tam E. Perry

http://orcid.org/0000-0002-8447-6115

Nancy Kusmaul

http://orcid.org/0000-0003-2278-8495

Cal J. Halvorsen

http://orcid.org/0000-0002-9184-633X

Disclosure statement

Tam E. Perry is the president, Nancy Kusmaul is the vice president, and Cal J. Halvorsen is the communications chair of the Association for Gerontology Education in Social Work (AGESW). AGESW is the official sponsor of the *Journal of Gerontological Social Work*.

Funding

The authors declare no sources of funding for this work.

References

Akiyama, M. J., Spaulding, A. C., & Rich, J. D. (2020). Flattening the curve for incarcerated populations—Covid-19 in jail and prisons. *New England Journal of Medicine, 382*(22), 2075–2077. https://doi.org/10.1056/NEJMp2005687

Archambault, D., Sanford, C., & Perry, T. (in press). Detroit's efforts to meet the needs of seniors: Macro responses to a crisis. *Journal of Gerontological Social Work*.

Association for Gerontology Education in Social Work. (2020). *Association for gerontology education in social work*. AGESW. https://agesw.org/

Centers for Disease Control and Prevention. (2020, June 25). *Older adults*. Coronavirus Disease 2019 (COVID-19). https://www.cdc.gov/coronavirus/2019-ncov/need-extra-precautions /older-adults.html

Council on Social Work Education. (2020). *Resources addressing coronavirus (COVID-19)*. CSWE. https://www.cswe.org/About-CSWE/Responding-to-Coronavirus

Ehrenfeld, J. M., & Harris, P. A. (2020, May 29). *Police brutality must stop*. American Medical Association. https://www.ama-assn.org/about/leadership/police-brutality-must-stop

Gramlich, J. (2020). *Black imprisonment rate in the U.S. has fallen by a third since 2006*. Pew Research Center. https://www.pewresearch.org/fact-tank/2020/05/06/black-imprisonment-rate-in-the-u-s-has-fallen-by-a-third-since-2006/

Grand Challenges for Social Work. (2020). *Grand challenges for social work*. https://grand challengesforsocialwork.org/

Halvorsen, C. J., & Yulikova, O. (2020a). Job training and so much more for low-income older adults: The senior community service employment program. *Clinical Social Work Journal, 48*(2), 223–229. https://doi.org/10.1007/s10615-019-00734-y

Halvorsen, C. J., & Yulikova, O. (2020b). Older workers in the time of COVID-19: The senior community service employment program and implications for social work. *Journal of Gerontological Social Work*, 1–12. Advance online publication. https://doi.org/10.1080/01634372.2020.1774832

Kusmaul, N., Bern-Klug, M., Heston-Mullins, J., Roberts, A. R., & Galambos, C. (2020). Nursing home social work during COVID-19. *Journal of Gerontological Social Work*. Advance Online Publication. https://doi.org/10.1080/01634372.2020.1787577

National Association of Social Workers. (2018). *Code of ethics: English*. https://www.socialwor kers.org/About/Ethics/Code-of-Ethics/Code-of-Ethics-English

National Association of Social Workers. (2020). *Coronavirus (COVID-19)*. NASW. https://www.socialworkers.org

National Center for Health Statistics. (2020, June 24). *Provisional death counts for coronavirus disease 2019 (COVID-19)*. Centers for Disease Control and Prevention. https://www.cdc.gov/nchs/nvss/vsrr/covid_weekly/index.htm

Rorai, V., & Perry, T. (2020). An innovative telephone outreach program to seniors in Detroit, a city facing dire consequences of COVID-19. *Journal of Gerontological Social Work.* Advance Online Publication. https://doi.org/10.1080/01634372.2020.1793254

Swinford, E., Galucia, N., & Morrow-Howell, N. (2020). Applying gerontological social work perspectives to the coronavirus pandemic. *Journal of Gerontological Social Work*, 1–11. Advance online publication. https://doi.org/10.1080/01634372.2020.1766628

The Impact of the COVID-19 Pandemic on Vulnerable Older Adults in the United States

Dear Editor,

Coronavirus disease 2019 (COVID-19) is an infectious disease reported to the World Health Organization (WHO) Country Office in China at the end of 2019 (World Health Organization [WHO], 2020a). As it continues to spread around the world, resulting in a pandemic, COVID-19 disproportionately impacts aging populations. In the United States, 8 out of 10 deaths have been those who are aged 65 years and older (Centers for Disease Control and Prevention [CDC], 2020b).

It is important to look back at how older adults have been susceptible to infectious disease and other respiratory conditions throughout history. The case-fatality ratio, measuring the "proportion of all people with a disease who will die from the disease", for SARS was estimated to be less than 1% in people aged 24 and younger whereas the ratio increased to more than 50% among older adults aged 65 and older across several countries (i.e., Canada, China, Hong Kong Special Administrative Region, Singapore, and Vietnam; WHO, 2003). Taking influenza as another example, people aged 65 and older represented 90% of influenza-related deaths and 50% to 70% of influenza-related hospitalizations during the influenza seasons spanning 2011 through 2015 in the United States (CDC, 2019). Similarly, COVID-19 exposes older adults to various added health and social risks.

The data shows differences in COVID-19 cases by age. As of the week ending May 16th, 2020, the cumulative COVID-19 incidence rate per 100,000 of the population aged 65+ was 214.4 in the United States. In contrast, people in other age groups had lower incidence rates per 100,000 of their respective populations compared to the older adult population (CDC, 2020c). It is possible that these numbers are underestimated due to factors such as lack of test availability, varying testing practices, and delays in reporting. In addition to older age, there are other socioeconomic factors that amplify the vulnerability of older adults during the COVID-19 pandemic era.

Gerontological social workers should pay extra attention to disadvantaged older adults, guided by the social determinants of health (SDH) conceptual framework. Vulnerable older adults include those who live in poverty, with a disability, and in social isolation. This letter provides background information on the SDH framework, identifies issues of heightened inequality, and offers recommendations on how our profession can support older adults experiencing additional disadvantages during the pandemic.

Issues of heightened inequality

Why are older adults at higher risk? Based on currently available information, old age, nursing home or long-term care facility living status, and medical condition status (e.g., chronic lung disease and serious heart conditions) are associated with higher risk of COVID-19 (CDC, 2020a).

The SDH conceptual framework offers insights to better understand how older adults may experience additional burden from the COVID-19 pandemic. The SDH conceptual framework presents the structural (e.g., socioeconomic and political factors) and intermediary determinants (e.g., material circumstances, behaviors, biological, and psychosocial factors) that influence equity in health and well-being (Solar & Irwin, 2010). According to this framework, several social justice issues arise from the COVID-19 pandemic.

Older adults living in poverty

Approximately 4.7 million older adults were in poverty in 2017 (Congressional Research Service, 2019). Living in poverty jeopardizes the health conditions of older adults during the COVID-19 pandemic because they may have limited access to alternative health care (e.g., telehealth) and may be experiencing food insecurity.

On March 27, 2020, the Coronavirus Aid, Relief, and Economic Security (CARES) Act was passed in the United States. The CARES Act provides support to workers, families, and businesses. As part of the CARES Act, the COVID-19 Telehealth Program supports eligible nonprofit and public health care providers with appropriate resources such as telecommunications services and necessary devices (Federal Communications Commission, 2020; U.S. Department of the Treasury, n.d.). Despite the effort to expand telehealth, older adults living in poverty may not have the appropriate means to utilize these services. Additionally, testing availability and other services may be limited.

Food insecurity is also a concern for older adults living in poverty. In 2018, there were 5.3 million older adults who experienced food insecurity in the United States (Gundersen & Ziliak, 2020). Due to the pandemic, disparities related to food insecurity may be worsened. Moreover, people of color and people with lower education levels disproportionately experience food insecurity (The Regents of the University of Michigan, 2020).

Older adults with disabilities

Older adults with disabilities are vulnerable to the COVID-19 pandemic. With the shortages of medical services and medication, people with disabilities face systematic challenges (American Psychological Association, 2020).

As an example, limited mobility is associated with frequent physical contact with care providers and family members to receive care, which puts people with mobility limitations at higher risk of exposure to contagious COVID-19 carriers. Also, maintaining good health and hygiene can be challenging with limited contact from health care providers. To overcome these hurdles, there are efforts to provide community-based support. San Francisco's Department of Disability and Aging Services (DAS) and community partners provide care support and food assistance by connecting older adults and people with disabilities with volunteers and paid care providers. DAS offers emergency on-call and short-term home care services regardless of Medi-Cal status. Food delivery, take-away meals, and grocery drop off programs provide access to food (City and County of San Francisco Human Services Agency, n.d.).

Social isolation

Social isolation, also referred to as loneliness (Elder & Retrum, 2012), is one of the social work grand challenges (Grand Challenges for Social Work, 2020a) and it impacts about 17% of older Americans aged 50+ (Elder & Retrum, 2012). The COVID-19 pandemic worsens the problem of isolation among older adults, engendering health and social consequences. Previous studies have highlighted the association between isolation and higher risks of negative health conditions such as heart disease, weakened immune systems, negative psychological well-being (e.g., anxiety and depression), cognitive decline, and premature mortality (Cornwell & Waite, 2009; National Institute on Aging, 2019; Valtorta & Hanratty, 2012). Isolated older adults are also at risk of elder abuse and financial scams. This means that isolation brings greater social challenges, such as additional costs for these health and social consequences.

Recommendations

To better support vulnerable older adults, the following section offers recommendations for each of the areas of structural and intermediary inequalities noted above.

Utilizing the SDH framework to identify the most vulnerable

Identifying older adults experiencing greater inequalities (e.g., those who live in poverty, with a disability, or in social isolation) during the pandemic can help social workers to enhance their support for them. The SDH conceptual framework presents structural determinants, such as socioeconomic position, social class, education, occupation, and income, as factors impacting health equity. Social workers should be involved in the care service decision-making process to address health-related barriers and to advocate for both short-term and long-term support. The role of gerontological social workers can be impactful in facilitating education and preparedness for the pandemic. In response to the ways that COVID-19 is impacting the community, social work educators serve as leaders in raising public awareness about vulnerable populations. For instance, from May through June, the University of Hawai'i at Mānoa Myron B. Thompson School of Social Work has been offering a free online webinar series on "COVID-19 and Vulnerable Communities". Webinar topics include the impact of the COVID-19 pandemic on older adults, racial and ethnic minorities, people with co-occurring disorders, and domestic violence victims. The twelve Grand Challenges for Social Work, including closing the health gap and eradicating social isolation, align well with the SDH conceptual framework (Grand Challenges for Social Work, 2020b). Thus, it is important for social workers to serve as leaders in identifying disadvantaged older adults.

Provide support for the most vulnerable

Systematically, older adults in poverty, with disabilities, or living in isolation, experience barriers in accessing health services. Even though telehealth helps to increase accessibility, we should be mindful that some older adults may lack technological resources and/or knowhow. Thus, it is vital to ensure accessible health services and to disseminate accurate information. For older adults with disabilities, their need for physical assistance puts them at higher risk of exposure to COVID-19 transmission. Home health care providers need to follow protocols such as having their temperature checked, washing their hands, and wearing masks. Social isolation interventions can be innovative. Smartphone applications such as social networking apps and communication apps can be used to alleviate loneliness and other negative health consequences (Banskota et al., 2020). Social workers should advocate for federal, state, and local assistance, and educate the public about available resources and evidence-based information.

Provide structural support to caregivers

Social workers must develop a long-term pandemic recovery plan for older adults that is guided by the SDH framework. Helping older adults during and after the pandemic requires support for the caregivers. To address the financial, physical, and psychological burdens of the pandemic, social workers need to advocate for federal, state, and local programs to support caregivers. It is critical to expand family support programs, such as the Families First Coronavirus Response Act (FFCRA). The FFCRA requires that employers allow employees to take emergency paid sick leave and emergency family medical leave, offering protections for caregivers and families due to the socioeconomic impact of the pandemic (U.S. Department of Labor, 2020a, 2020b). To systematically address the needs of older adults and their families, social workers must continue to advocate for policy changes.

To protect older adults during the COVID-19 pandemic, local to national level efforts are needed that recognize their vulnerability. Gerontological social workers and health care professionals need to promote COVID-19 prevention strategies, offer health education, and advocate for government support. These efforts can help in reaching out to marginalized older adults and supporting those who may be suffering from issues such as COVID-19 symptoms, health complications, social isolation, and other disparities. We urgently need to expand our knowledge on health inequalities and to increase support for addressing them. During the pandemic, the SDH framework reminds us that health is linked to complex social factors. The current knowledge suggests innovative ways to improve health outcomes and to alleviate the negative impacts of the pandemic for socially disadvantaged older adults. The role of gerontological social workers is critical in addressing structural challenges. The global response to the pandemic can be strengthened by applying the SDH framework.

Yeonjung Jane Lee

References

American Psychological Association. (2020). *Fighting inequity in the face of COVID-19*. https://www.apa.org/monitor/2020/06/covid-fighting-inequity

Banskota, S., Healy, M., & Goldberg, E. M. (2020). 15 smartphone Apps for older adults to use while in isolation during the COVID-19 pandemic. *Western Journal of Emergency Medicine: Integrating Emergency Care with Population Health, 21*(3), 514–525. https://doi.org/10.5811/westjem.2020.4.47372

Centers for Disease Control and Prevention. (2019). *Influenza (Flu). Study shows hospitalization rates and risk of death from seasonal flu increase with age among people 65 years and older*. https://www.cdc.gov/flu/spotlights/2018-2019/hopitalization-rates-older.html

Centers for Disease Control and Prevention. (2020a). *Coronavirus disease 2019 (COVID-19). Groups at higher risk for severe illness*. https://www.cdc.gov/coronavirus/2019-ncov/need-extra-precautions/groups-at-higher-risk.html

Centers for Disease Control and Prevention. (2020b). *Coronavirus Disease 2019 (COVID-19).* Older Adults. https://www.cdc.gov/coronavirus/2019-ncov/need-extra-precautions/older-adults.html

Centers for Disease Control and Prevention. (2020c). *COVID-NET: COVID-19-Associated Hospitalization Surveillance Network, Centers for Disease Control and Prevention.* https://gis.cdc.gov/grasp/covidnet/COVID19_3.html

City and County of San Francisco Human Services Agency. (n.d.). *COVID-19 updates for older adults and people with disabilities.* https://www.sfhsa.org/services/protection-safety/emergency-preparedness-and-assistance/hsa-coronavirus-updates/covid-19

Congressional Research Service. (2019). *Poverty among Americans aged 65 and older.* https://fas.org/sgp/crs/misc/R45791.pdf

Cornwell, E. Y., & Waite, L. J. (2009). Social disconnectedness, perceived isolation, and health among older adults. *Journal of Health and Social Behavior, 50*(1), 31–48. https://doi.org/10.1177/002214650905000103

Elder, K., & Retrum, J. (2012). *Framework for isolation in adults over 50.* https://www.aarp.org/content/dam/aarp/aarp_foundation/2012_PDFs/AARP-Foundation-Isolation-Framework-Report.pdf

Federal Communications Commission (2020). *COVID-19 telehealth program.* https://www.fcc.gov/covid-19-telehealth-program

Grand Challenges for Social Work. (2020a). *Eradicate social isolation.* https://grandchallengesforsocialwork.org/eradicate-social-isolation/

Grand Challenges for Social Work (2020b). *Grand challenges for social work.* https://grandchallengesforsocialwork.org/

Gundersen, C., & Ziliak, J. (2020). *The state of senior hunger in America 2018: An annual report.* Report submitted to Feeding America. https://www.feedingamerica.org/research/senior-hunger-research/senior

National Institute on Aging. (2019). *Social isolation, loneliness in older people pose health risks.* https://www.nia.nih.gov/news/social-isolation-loneliness-older-people-pose-health-risks

The Regents of the University of Michigan. (2020). *Even before COVID-19, many adults over 50 lacked stable food supply, didn't use assistance.* https://news.umich.edu/even-before-covid-19-many-adults-over-50-lacked-stable-food-supply-didnt-use-assistance/

Solar, O., & Irwin, A. (2010). A conceptual framework for action on the social determinants of health. Retrieved from Social Determinants of Health Discussion Paper 2 (Policy and Practice). https://www.who.int/sdhconference/resources/ConceptualframeworkforactiononSDH_eng.pdf

U.S. Department of Labor. (2020a). *Families first coronavirus response act: Employee paid leave rights.* https://www.dol.gov/agencies/whd/pandemic/ffcra-employee-paid-leave

U.S. Department of Labor. (2020b). *COVID-19 and the American workplace.* https://www.dol.gov/agencies/whd/pandemic

U.S. Department of the Treasury. (n.d.). *The CARES act works for all Americans.* https://home.treasury.gov/policy-issues/cares

Valtorta, N., & Hanratty, B. (2012). Loneliness, isolation and the health of older adults: Do we need a new research agenda? *Journal of the Royal Society of Medicine, 105*(12), 518–522. https://doi.org/10.1258/jrsm.2012.120128

World Health Organization. (2003). *Emergencies preparedness, response. Update 49 - SARS case fatality ratio, incubation period.* https://www.who.int/csr/sarsarchive/2003_05_07a/en/

World Health Organization. (2020a). *Rolling updates on coronavirus disease (COVID-19).* https://www.who.int/emergencies/diseases/novel-coronavirus-2019/events-as-they-happen

Social Work Values in Action during COVID-19

Dear Editor

COVID-19 has ravaged through the lives of individuals, families, communities, and societies and, in the process, exacerbated existing vulnerabilities, oppression, and poverty among our most at-risk older adults. Social workers, guided by values and ethics, are counteracting these ailments in society, concentrating on protecting the most vulnerable. As described in the guiding Code of Ethics and Values, the primary mission of social work, "is to enhance human well-being and help meet the basic human needs of all people, with particular attention to the needs and empowerment of people who are vulnerable, oppressed, and living in poverty" (National Association of Social Workers [NASW], 2017, para. 1). Social workers are demonstrating heroic work on the frontlines. Here we describe the impact of COVID-19 on older adults and highlight the current role of the practicing social worker putting these values in action during COVID-19.

Older adults are at a significantly higher risk for COVID-19 (Centers for Disease Control and Prevention [CDC], 2020a). Eight out of 10 deaths reported have been among adults who are aged 65 years and above (Centers for Disease Control and Prevention [CDC], 2020a), with a reported mortality rate of approximately 15% (Wu & McGoogan, 2020). These devastating consequences of COVID-19 are impacting older adults, family, and friends. Older adults living independently relying on various community services may now be faced with an inability to meet their basic needs (e.g., housing and nutrition). Aging adults watching the news are witnessing deaths; family members who have lost a loved one are unable to arrange or attend funeral services, and aging family members displaced are unable to connect with those most important to them, resulting in loss and grief in isolation.

Similarly, and perhaps more so, older adults in senior living facilities are aggressively impacted by COVID-19. Nursing facilities are home to the most at-risk seniors, with over 7,000 residents having died as a direct result of this pandemic (Bunis, 2020). Residents who have not contracted COVID-19 may have witnessed a roommate or friend succumb to this virus. Residents with family are now faced with extreme isolation, as restrictions to visitation were implemented. Likewise, family members may be faced with an extreme sense of guilt and loss of placing their loved one in a nursing home (Hagen, 2001). The reduction in staff and key personnel due to the risks associated with COVID-19, while a practical response to the current pandemic, may impact resident well-being. These relationships between staff and residents are found to be important

(Roberts, 2018), and staff turnover has a detrimental impact on resident overall wellness (Plaku-Alakbarova et al., 2018).

It is also necessary to report the uptick in xenophobia and racism related to the current pandemic. Asians Americans and Pacific Islanders are experiencing stigma and discrimination (Centers for Disease Control and Prevention [CDC], 2020a). This population is being subjected to rejection, social avoidance, denial of healthcare, housing, and even physical violence (Centers for Disease Control and Prevention [CDC], 2020a). Racism impacts health, mental health, and overall well-being (Cramer & Smith McElveen, 2003). During this time, there is a dedicated demonstration of social work values in action by practicing social workers (National Association of Social Workers [NASW], 2017):

- **Social Justice**: Social workers (SWs) are on the frontlines challenging social injustices. SWs are working to promote cultural sensitivity within communities, increase knowledge, and educate the public on marginalized populations (Wilson, 2020). SWs are connecting underserved populations to care, including health and behavioral health services (NASW, 2016). Practitioners are gathering resources on culturally adapted behavioral interventions to bridge the gap between service use and intervention outcomes among historically marginalized and oppressed populations (CSWE, n.d.).
- **Importance of Human Relationships**: For home-bound older adults, SWs are delivering hot meals regularly through programs such as Meals on Wheels (MOW). These interactions between MOW and the clients are more than just food; research shows that clients derive social bonds and establish social relationships with MOW personnel that are strengthened over time (Thomas et al., 2020). Additional efforts are being made to promote social connection through alternative modes, such as telephone friendship hotlines.
- **Integrity**: SWs and senior advocacy groups are initiating virtual visitation programs to mitigate the psychological distress such as depression and social isolation (Canady, 2020) and to maintain connections within the community (National Council on Aging [NCOA], 2020). SWs are serving seniors through HIPAA-compliant, confidential, trustworthy telehealth modalities focusing attention on loss and grief (McCarty & Clancy, 2002).
- **Dignity and Worth of the Individual**: Long-term care SWs are advocating for and ensuring each resident attains their highest level of psychosocial well-being possible (Bern-Klug et al., 2009). Given the current pandemic, these SWs are going above and beyond to address the social- and emotional- needs of nursing home residents and family members. SWs are engaging in discharge planning, working to navigate the ever-

complex and disjointed health care delivery system as hospitals respond to the surge in COVID-19 cases.

- **Competence**: Aging focused SWs are educating and supporting staff within communities and senior living facilities. SWs are promoting alternative treatment methods to reduce depression, isolation, and loneliness through social interaction via various modes of communication such as the internet and other devices (Tsai et al., 2017). Even more, SWs are developing alternative programs to the traditional models of care (e.g., senior centers), while promoting prevention education for aging community members.

- **Service**: Through each of these practices, SWs are leveraging practice skills of engagement and community connection to rally others to serve this at-risk population. Example efforts include organizing expansive food pantry collections at local senior centers, developing neighborhood grocery delivery programs to vulnerable older adults, and compiling web-based resources with lists for assistance in benefits, utilities, transportation, and mental health services (NCOA, 2020).

While this is not complete description of the SWs response in this time of crisis, it is clear that the current pandemic is "undoubtedly changing the way we live" (Weir, 2020). Even after this crisis comes to an end, a wider spectrum of older adults living with children and persons with disabilities, mainly those of low socioeconomic status, will continually need the help of practicing SWs. In this context, the social work profession, guided by ethics and values, is stepping up to uniquely engage in issues concerning human rights, well-being, and social equity for all older adults.

Sincerely,

Vivian J. Miller and HeeSoon Lee

ⓘ http://orcid.org/0000-0003-2030-862X

References

Bern-Klug, M., Kramer, K. W. O., Chan, G., Kane, R., Dorfman, L. T., & Saunders, J. (2009). Characteristics of nursing home social services directors: How common is a degree in social work? *Journal of the American Medical Directors Association, 10*(1), 36–44. https://doi.org/10.1016/j.jamda.2008.06.011

Bunis, D. (2020). Nursing homes ordered to disclose COVID-19 cases, deaths. AARP. Retrieved from https://www.aarp.org/caregiving/health/info-2020/nursing-homes-to-publicly-disclose-coronavirus.html

Canady, V. A. (2020). COVID-19 outbreak represents a new way of mental health service delivery. *Mental Health Weekly*, *30*(12), 1–4. https://doi-org.ezproxy.bgsu.edu/10.1002/mhw.32282

Centers for Disease Control and Prevention [CDC]. (2020a). *Older adults.* CDC/Coronavirus Disease 2019 (COVID-19). Centers for Disease Control and Prevention. Retrieved from https://www.cdc.gov/coronavirus/2019-ncov/need-extra-precautions/older-adults.html

Council on Social Work Education [CSWE]. (n.d.) Cultural adaptation of behavioral interventions: Annotated bibliography. Council on Social Work Education. Retrieved from https://www.cswe.org/Centers-Initiatives/Centers/Center-for-Diversity/Curriculum-Resources/Resources-for-Practice-with-Diverse-Communities/Cultural-Adaptation-of-Behavioral-Interventions

Cramer, D. N., & Smith McElveen, J. (2003). Undoing racism in social work practice. *Race, Gender, & Class*, *10*(2), 41–57. https://www.jstor.org/stable/41675072

Hagen, B. (2001). Nursing home placement: factors affecting caregivers' decisions to place family members with dementia. *Journal of Gerontological Nursing.*, *27*(2), 44–53. https://doi.org/10.3928/0098-9134-20010201-14

McCarty, D., & Clancy, C. (2002). Telehealth: Implications for social work practice. *Social Work*, *47*(2), 153–161. https://doi.org/10.1093/sw/47.2.153

National Association of Social Workers [NASW]. (2016). *NASW practice standards for social work practice in health care settings*. National Association of Social Workers.Retrieved from https://www.socialworkers.org/LinkClick.aspx?fileticket=fFnsRHX-4HE%3d&portalid=0

National Association of Social Workers [NASW]. (2017). *Code of Ethics*. National Association of Social Workers. Retrieved from https://www.socialworkers.org/about/ethics/code-of-ethics/code-of-ethics-english

National Council on Aging [NCOA]. (2020). *COVID resources for older adults and caregivers*. National Council on Aging. Retrieved from https://www.ncoa.org/covid-19/covid-19-resources-for-older-adults/

Plaku-Alakbarova, B., Punnett, L., Gore, R. J., & Team, P. R. (2018). Nursing home employee and resident satisfaction and resident care outcomes. *Safety and Health at Work*, *9*(4), 408–415. https://doi.org/10.1016/j.shaw.2017.12.002

Roberts, T. J. (2018). Nursing home resident relationship types: What supports close relationships with peers & staff? *Journal of Clinical Nursing*, *27*(23–24), 4361–4372. https://doi.org/10.1111/jocn.14554

Thomas, K. S., Gadbois, E. A., Shield, R. R., Akobundu, U., Morris, A. M., & Dosa, D. M. (2020). "It's Not Just a Simple Meal. It's So Much More": Interactions Between Meals on Wheels Clients and Drivers. *Journal of Applied Gerontology*, *39*(2), 151–158. https://doi.org/10.1177/0733464818820226

Tsai, T.-H., Chang, H.-T., Chen, Y.-J., Chang, Y.-S., & Xia, F. (2017). Determinants of user acceptance of a specific social platform for older adults: An empirical examination of user interface characteristics and behavioral intention. *PLoS ONE*, *12*(8), e0180102. https://doi.org/10.1371/journal.pone.0180102

Weir, K. (2020). *Grief and COVID-19: Saying goodbye in the age of physical distancing*. American Psychological Association. Retrieved from https://www.apa.org/topics/covid-19/grief-distance

Wilson, M. (2020). *Implications of Coronavirus (COVID-19) for America's Vulnerable and Marginalized Populations*. Social Justice Brief. Retrieved from https://www.socialworkers.org/LinkClick.aspx?fileticket=U7tEKlRldOU%3D&portalid=0

Wu, J., & McGoogan, J. M. (2020). Characteristics of and important lessons from the coronavirus disease 2019 (COVID-19) outbreak in China: Summary of a report of 72 314 cases from the chinese center for disease control and prevention. *JAMA*, *323*(13), 1239–1242. https://doi.org/10.1001/jama.2020.2648

COVID-19 and Older Adults: The Time for Gerontology-Curriculum across Social Work Programs is Now!

Dear Editor-in-Chief,

Older adulthood involves increased risk for falls, chronic diseases (e.g., cardiovascular disease, respiratory illness, diabetes), and changes in physical mobility. Compounding these natural and unnatural consequences of the aging process, the current COVID-19 pandemic has placed older adults at increased risk for serious disease and death (Centers for Disease Control and Prevention [CDC], 2020a). Current statistics report that as many as eight out of 10 COVID-19 deaths in the United States (U.S.) have been persons aged 65 and older (Centers for Disease Control and Prevention [CDC], 2020b).

In addition to practicing in the community, gerontological social workers practice in senior living facilities and medical settings; these include assisted living facilities (ALFs), nursing homes (NHs), and hospitals. These settings have a high proportion of older residents and patients and have been epicenters to especially high rates of COVID-19 cases and deaths. Over 800,000 older adults reside in ALFs across the U.S., and this population is at significant risk for COVID-19 (Kaiser Health News [KHN], 2020). In April, there were over 700 cases of COVID-19 across ALFs reported (Kaiser Health News [KHN], 2020), and this number has only grown since. Nursing home (NH) residents, especially long-term care residents who live in NHs permanently due to requiring 24-hour level of care (as opposed to short-term skilled nursing residents), are highly vulnerable to COVID-19. The University of Minnesota [UMN], 2020 cites that 40% of all virus-related deaths have taken place in a NH. This estimates that, since March, approximately 450 older adult NH residents have died per day across the U.S., and this is likely an underestimate (University of Minnesota [UMN], 2020). Lastly, hospitals represent the first and/or last point of contact for older adults experiencing symptoms of COVID-19. A recent study (Cummings et al., 2020) published findings from a New York hospital where the average length of stay was three days before an older adult died as a result of the virus.

Assisted living facility social workers offer counseling, resource coordination, and family support services (Vinton, 2008). Nursing home social workers coordinate care, arrange family visitation, educate staff, and ensure each resident attains their highest level of psychosocial well-being possible (National Association of Social Workers [NASW], 2003). Medical/hospital social workers advocate for patients, conduct psychosocial assessments, coordinate resources, and engage in discharge planning, among other tasks (Gibelman, 1995; Holliman et al., 2001). A shortage of gerontology-trained social workers has been reported for over a decade (Beltran & Miller, 2019) and the latest research identifying social work practice areas reports that less than 10% of licensed social workers practice in the field of aging (Lustig, 2013; Whitaker et al., 2006 in Beltran & Miller, 2019).

All social workers are likely to encounter older clients at various points in their careers regardless of their specialization, as evidenced by the settings discussed above where social workers practice (i.e., NHs, ALFs, hospitals) and where older adults, given the aging process and multiple chronic conditions, are a key client population. As the present global emergency highlights, there is an urgent need for social work programs to prepare all rising social workers to work with older clients, undergraduate and graduate-level alike. Social work programs must engage in deliberate efforts to increase the number of program graduates devoted to practicing in gerontology. Furthermore, regardless of primary specialization, all social workers must have competency working with older clients and be prepared to support the unique needs of older adults that surface in emergency situations such as this pandemic (Kusmaul et al., 2018).

There is a need for the Council on Social Work Education (CSWE) to strengthen the emphasis on age within its educational policy and standards (CSWE, 2015). Currently, age is only mentioned twice within the EPAS document; it is listed as a dimension of the diversity competency. Age is not covered equitably across the curriculum, and the number of social work program graduates that specialize in gerontology remains low compared to other specializations (Lee, 2019). CSWE's Gero-Ed Center, an aging-specific social work initiative to infuse gerontology content throughout the curriculum, has not received any funding since 2015 (Council on Social Work Education [CSWE], n.d.). Re-funding this initiative or reestablishing efforts to infuse gerontology content throughout the curriculum needs to be a renewed priority. Social workers are uniquely positioned to help address the psychosocial, spiritual, and cultural needs and preferences of older adults. Workforce developments are required now, in order to ensure the growing older adult population is supported in their last stage of life.

Sincerely,

Susanny J. Beltran

Vivian J. Miller

http://orcid.org/0000-0003-2030-862X

Disclosure statement

The authors have no disclosures.

References

Beltran, S. J., & Miller, V. J. (2019). Breaking Out of the Silo: A Systematic Review of University-Level Gerontological Curricula in Social Work and Nursing Programs. *Journal of Social Work Education*, 1-26. doi:10.1080/10437797.2019.1656689

Centers for Disease Control and Prevention [CDC]. (2020a). *Older adults*. Centers for Disease Control and Prevention. https://www.cdc.gov/coronavirus/2019-ncov/need-extra-precautions/older-adults.html

Centers for Disease Control and Prevention [CDC]. (2020b). *Severe outcomes among patients with coronavirus disease 2019 (COVID-2019) – United States, February 12-March 16, 2020*. Morbidity and Mortality Weekly Report. http://www.ecie.com.ar/images/paginas/COVID-19/4MMWR-Severe_Outcomes_Among_Patients_with_Coronavirus_Disease_2019_COVID-19-United_States_February_12-March_16_2020.pdf

Council on Social Work Education (CSWE). (2015). *Educational policy and accreditation standards*. https://www.cswe.org/getattachment/Accreditation/Accreditation-Process/2015-EPAS/2015EPAS_Web_FINAL.pdf.aspx

Council on Social Work Education (CSWE). (n.d.). *About the gero-ed center*. https://www.cswe.org/Centers-Initiatives/Centers/Gero-Ed-Center/About

Cummings, M. J., Baldwin, M. R., O'Donnell, M. R., Meyer, B. J., Balough, E. M., Aaron, J. G., Claassen, J., Rabbani, L. E., Hastie, J., Hochman, B. R., Salazar-Schicchi, J., Yip, N. H., Brodie, D., O'Donnell, M. R., & Abrams, D. (2020). Epidemiology, clinical course, and outcomes of critically ill adults with COVID-19 in New York City: A prospective cohort study. *The Lancet*, 395(10239), 1763–1770. https://doi.org/10.1016/S0140-6736(20)31189-2

Gibelman, M. (1995). *What social workers do* (Vol. 131). NASW Press.

Holliman, D. C., Dziegielewsk, S. F., & Datta, P. (2001). Discharge planning and social work practice. *Social Work in Health Care*, 32(3), 1–19. https://doi.org/10.1300/J010v32n03_01

Kaiser Health News [KHN]. (2020). *COVID-19 crisis threatens beleaguered assisted living industry*. Kaiser Health News. https://khn.org/news/covid-19-crisis-threatens-beleaguered-assisted-living-industry/

Kusmaul, N., Gibson, A., & Leedahl, S. N. (2018). Gerontological social work roles in disaster preparedness and response. *Journal of Gerontological Social Work*, 61(7), 692–696. https://doi.org/10.1080/01634372.2018.1510455

Lee, K. (2019). Reflections and prospects of the gerontological social work training and education: The AGESW pre-dissertation fellows program. *Journal of Gerontological Social Work*, 62(8), 867–872. https://doi.org/10.1080/01634372.2019.1686674

Lustig, T. A. (2013). *Statement before the commission on long term care*. http://ltccommission.org/ltccommission/wp-content/uploads/2013/12/Tracy-Lustig

National Association of Social Workers [NASW]. (2003). *NASW standards for social work services in long-term care facilities*. National Association of Social Workers. https://www.socialworkers.org/LinkClick.aspx?fileticket=cwW7lzBfYxg%3D&portalid=0

University of Minnesota [UMN]. (2020). *Nursing homes site 40% of US COVID-19 related deaths*. Center for Infectious Disease Research and Policy. https://www.cidrap.umn.edu/news-perspective/2020/06/nursing-homes-site-40-us-covid-19-deaths

Vinton, L. (2008). Perceptions of the need for social work in assisted living. *Journal of Social Work in Long-term Care*, 3(1), 85–100. https://doi.org/10.1300/J181v03n01_07

Whitaker, T., Weismiller, T., & Clark, E. (2006). *Assuring the sufficiency of a frontline workforce: A national study of licensed social workers*. National Association of Social Workers.

They are Essential Workers Now, and Should Continue to Be: Social Workers and Home Health Care Workers during COVID-19 and Beyond

Dear Editor,

Although much has been said over the past few months about the selfless dedication of frontline healthcare workers during the Coronavirus (COVID-19) pandemic, this deserved recognition stands in stark contrast to the decades of neglect that some members of this workforce have historically endured. That is, while social workers and home health care workers often serve as the backbone of our social service delivery and healthcare systems, they have been and continue to be, seldom seen, heard, or valued. Social workers, despite their roles in hospitals and nursing homes, are not being recognized as "essential" workers (Lipe, 2020). Similarly, home health care workers, despite caring for older adults with those with disabilities, functional deficits, and medical comorbidities, are invisible essential workers in many states during COVID-19.

Currently, 2.3 million workers provide hands-on personal assistance and health care support to 8.3 older adults in the home and community-based settings (Campbell, 2017). These workers are essential to the successful completion of fundamental activities of daily living (ADLs) and instrumental ADLs (IADLs). Additionally, they aid with medically-oriented tasks such as reminding patients to take medications, accompanying them to health care visits, and taking vital signs. Beyond that, they provide emotional support and companionship. Social workers know and understand the value of these workers, since the independence of their clients is contingent on having their support (Reckrey et al., 2019; Sterling & Shaw, 2019).

Yet despite being integral to patient and community care, these workers – who are mostly middle-age women from racial, ethnic and/or immigrant communities – experience daily hardships. As social workers know, they work long hours, often for multiple agencies, earn minimum wages, and have few opportunities for career advancement. According to data from PHI, home health care workers earn a median hourly wage of 11.52 USD and an annual salary of 16,200 USD (Workforce Data Center, 2017). Currently, more than half rely on some form of public assistance. These conditions have led to high turnover rates and workforce shortages, which are likely to be exacerbated during COVID-19 if the workforce is not better supported.

As COVID-19 overwhelms our healthcare and social service systems, and more older adults are asked to manage their symptoms at home, the role and importance of community-based supports, especially home health care workers, will become increasingly important for patients. Yet, because home health care workers are in close contact with frail, elderly, and medically complex clients, they are at an increased risk of exposure to COVID-19. This puts their own health and that of their families' in jeopardy. Home health care workers in many areas also face shortages of personal protective equipment (PPE), which further increases transmission risk. Unlike other healthcare workers, taking sick leave is not always an option for this group. Beyond losing their own wages, a recent survey by PHI found that 66% of workers are concerned that there won't be enough workers to replace them if they need to take time off or leave their existing jobs due to COVID-19 (Scales, 2020). All told, the impact of COVID-19 may be devastating for direct care workers and their clients, unless serious action is taken.

Social workers are key players in interdisciplinary healthcare and serve as a critical link to home health care workers by recommending and approving services for clients, managing and training workers, and advocating for client-centered supports. *So what can they do for workers during COVID-19?* First, social workers can serve as advocates for home health care workers to receive training on COVID-19 and infection control practices from health systems, employers, and government agencies. Evidence suggest that high quality training improves workers' preparedness and confidence, as well as the quality of care they deliver (Guerrero et al., 2019). Second, technology needs to be leveraged to meet workers' training needs during COVID, when social distancing is necessary. With physical distancing mandates, social workers can provide or advocate that training be conducted remotely, online, by phone or through information mailings to ensure the safety of both the workers and their clients. Third, home health care workers need supplies. Just as hospitals are scrambling to meet daily PPE requirements, so are community based organizations and social service agencies. Yet, unlike large hospitals, these agencies do not have the same buying power or bargaining ability. Therefore, serious advocacy is necessary for both local and state agencies, home care associations, and healthcare worker unions – and social workers can help. Lastly, policies are needed to better support these workers. COVID-19 is a fitting time to revisit previous calls for a healthcare and employment model that recognizes, rewards, and respects interdisciplinary care, and highlights the role of home health and direct care workers' contribution to the health, safety, and quality of life of older adults and those with chronic conditions and disabilities. In particular, policies are needed that at the very least, provide workers with living wages and benefits, including paid sick leave, health insurance, and retirement contributions. Ideally, organizations should move away from an approach that relies on temporary and contingent workers. Social workers can serve as advocates for these and other policies that are supportive of these workers and their clients.

As community spread of COVID-19 continues, and as more Americans shelter in place, the burden of care will be increasingly placed on home health and direct care workers, a group of front-line caregivers that has historically been overlooked and undervalued by the healthcare system and society at large. *Now is the time to change this.* Now is the time for increased awareness and advocacy by the social work community that understands the value and needs of community-based care. Home health care workers need far more than our acknowledgment and appreciation. They need policies that improve training, provide equipment, ensure stable, good paying, and high-quality jobs so they can continue to care for our communities and loved ones safely and securely. Our social work values and ethics demand we do this for our older adults now, and into the future.

Lourdes R. Guerrero

ⓘ http://orcid.org/0000-0003-4208-4786

Ariel C. Avgar

Erica Phillips and Madeline R. Sterling

References

Campbell, S. (2017). *US home care workers: key facts.* PHI national.

Guerrero, L. R., Eldridge, C., & Tan, Z. S. (2019). Competency-based training for in-home supportive services providers of consumers with ADRD. *Gerontology & Geriatrics Education,* 41(1), 121–132. https://doi.org/10.1080/02701960.2019.1658579

Lipe, L. (2020, May 11). *Social workers are essential workers.* The New Social Worker. Retrieved May 23, 2020, from https://www.socialworker.com/feature-articles/practice/social-workers-essential-workers/

Reckrey, J. M., Tsui, E. K., Morrison, R. S., Geduldig, E. T., Stone, R. I., Ornstein, K. A., & Federman, A. D. (2019). Beyond functional support: The range of health-related tasks performed in the home by paid caregivers in New York. *Health Affairs,* 38(6), 927–933. https://doi.org/10.1377/hlthaff.2019.00004

Scales, K. (2020, April 6). *We surveyed our stakeholders on COVID-19.* Here's What We Learned. PHI National. Retrieved May 23, 2020, from https://phinational.org/we-surveyed-our-stakeholders-on-covid-19-heres-what-we-learned/

Sterling, M. R., & Shaw, A. L. (2019). Sharing the care—A patient and her caregivers. *JAMA Internal Medicine,* 179(12), 1617. https://doi.org/10.1001/jamainternmed.2019.4231

Workforce Data Center. (2017, September 6). Retrieved May 23, 2020, from https://phinational.org/policy-research/workforce-data-center/

A Reflection of and Charge to Gerontological Social Work: Past Pandemics and the Current COVID-19 Crisis

Dear Editor-in-Chief,

Despite COVID-19 being a novel experience, it is neither the first example of, nor the first instance where, the social work profession has played a significant role. Human history is punctuated by tragedy, often troubled by social barriers influencing the depth and breadth of response. It is here where social workers have, historically, been on the frontlines, responding to pandemics and emergency situations. The current global health crisis provides opportunity to reflect on prior social work responses to prior pandemic situations and serves to inform future research and practice for vulnerable older adults.

The following examples elucidate the gravity of pandemics similar to COVID-19:

Influenza pandemic of 1918

The Influenza Pandemic of 1918–1920 was a global tragedy, bringing illness to over one-third of the world's population. Though 20–50 million persons perished from the "Great Flu," even more experienced loss and hardship, secondary to economic and social structures already in the throes from the end of World War I. Kerson (1979) provided a retrospective assessment of social work response to the emergent needs of the broad swath of persons and communities recovering from assaults, secondary to the Influenza of 1918, including older persons and persons living with chronic illness, economic insecurity, overburdened healthcare organizations, widespread unemployment, and trauma. This response set the stage for professional social work response to emergent events.

Acquired Immunodeficiency Syndrome (AIDS) & Human Immunodeficiency Virus HIV

AIDS was recognized as a new disease in 1981, and mortality rate by 1983 was 39% (Jaffe et al., 1983). As we approach the fourth decade of the HIV/AIDS pandemic, approximately 65 million infections and 25 million deaths have been recorded (Centers for Disease Control (CDC), 1981). In addition, approximately 38 million people were living with HIV as of 2018. Though antiretroviral therapies extend life expectancy significantly (Global, 2019), men who have sex with men and intravenous drug users, and other stigmatized persons bear both the high risk of infection and greater lack of access to care. Almost half of all HIV+ patients in the U.S. are over age 50 (Levy-Dweck, 2005). Gerontological social workers (GSWs) support patients with HIV/AIDS, applying a biopsychosocial approach to prevention, education, testing, intervention, and advocacy efforts (Mantell et al., 1989; National Association of Social Workers (NASW), 2015), and will continue to address the persistent needs of this global epidemic.

SARS

From November 2002 to late 2003, the spread of SARS extended across 33 countries, with a 10–15% mortality rate (Rowlands, 2007), with older adults identified as a high-risk group, due to vulnerabilities exacerbated by health conditions and other social factors. During SARS, GSWs identified uncertainty about frequent changes to infection control policies, anxiety, fear of infecting friends and family, and stigmatization and rejection because of hospital work in their communities as issues that immediately impacted their lives (Bai et al., 2004). Here, social workers were, again, on the frontline of emergency response services in several countries, with GSWs among the multidisciplinary staff trained in emergency behaviors protocols, providing key emergency management and recovery tasks (Rowlands, 2007).

Parnett and Rothstein (2018) identified "hubris, isolationism, and distrust" as the greatest challenges to social health and social welfare (p. 1435). These continue to create and maintain social barriers for vulnerable persons, often dismissed, othered, or suggested as unworthy. As COVID-19 ravages the lives of older adults, care providers, families, and communities at-large, we remain on the frontlines, fighting for the dignity and worth of vulnerable community members, continuing to navigate the ever-changing and complex health care systems for aging patients and clients. Drawing on our responses to prior epidemics, it is clear that we have and will continue to advocate, empower, and serve our most vulnerable, by:

- Providing key analyses of the intersection of stress, trauma, and multiple disadvantages.
- Supporting COVID-19 patients, as well as other individuals associated with them (i.e., relatives, health care staff).
- Developing GSW initiatives to define best practices in emergency responses, including use of telehealth.
- Advocating for policies to prepare and proactively address needs in future crises.
- Continuing research efforts with dedicated attention to marginalized, at-risk older adults who are sheltering in place at home in the community and those isolated in congregate living situations (e.g., nursing homes).

We are here, we will continue our efforts to mitigate and lessen complex problems experienced during these – and future – unprecedented times, forging ahead to fight for and enhance the collective well-being of communities facing trials, tribulations, and trauma brought by emergencies and disasters.

Sincerely,

Tyrone C. Hamler

Sara J. English

Susanny J. Beltran

Vivian J. Miller

ⓘ http://orcid.org/0000-0003-2030-862X

References

Bai, Y., Lin, C. C., Lin, C. Y., Chen, J. Y., Chue, C. M., & Chou, P. (2004). Survey of stress reactions among health care workers involved with the SARS outbreak. *Psychiatric Services*, *55*(9), 1055–1057. https://doi.org/10.1176/appi.ps.55.9.1055

Centers for Disease Control (CDC). (1981). Kaposi's sarcoma and Pneumocystis pneumonia among homosexual men–New York City and California. *Morbidity and Mortality Weekly Report*, *30*(25), 305. https://doi.org/10.1038/s41598-019-51320-8

Global, H. I. V. (2019). *AIDS statistics—2018 fact sheet*. https://www.unaids.org/sites/default/files/media_asset/UNAIDS_FactSheet_en.pdf

Jaffe, H. W., Bregman, D. J., & Selik, R. M. (1983). Acquired immune deficiency syndrome in the United States: The first 1,000 cases. *Journal of Infectious Diseases*, *148*(2), 339–345. https://doi.org/10.1093/infdis/148.2.339

Kerson, T. S. (1979). Sixty years ago: Hospital social work in 1918. *Social Work in Healthcare*, *4*(3), 331–343. https://doi.org/10.1300/J010v04n03_08

Levy-Dweck, S. (2005). HIV/AIDS fifty and older: A hidden and growing population. *Journal of Gerontological Social Work*, *46*(2), 37–50. https://doi.org/10.1300/J083v46n02_04

Mantell, J. E., Shulman, L. C., Belmont, M. F., & Spivak, H. B. (1989). Social workers respond to the AIDS epidemic in an acute care hospital. *Health & Social Work*, *14*(1), 41–51. https://doi.org/10.1093/hsw/14.1.41

National Association of Social Workers (NASW). (2015). *Social work practice: Engaging individuals, communities, and systems in support of the national HIV/AIDS strategy*. www.socialworkers.org/LinkClick.aspx?fileticket=nNElZxf3cHc%3d&portalid=0

Parnett, W. E., & Rothstein, M. A. (2018). The 1918 influenza epidemic: Lessons learned and not - Introduction to the special section. *American Journal of Public Health*, *108*(11), 1435–1436. https://doi.org/10.2105/AJPH.2018.304695

Rowlands, A. (2007). Medical social work practice and SARS in Singapore. *Social Work in Health Care*, *45*(3), 57–83. https://doi.org/10.1300/J010v45n03_04

Part III

COVID-19 and Social Work
with Diverse Groups

The Disproportionate Impact of COVID-19 on Minority Groups: A Social Justice Concern

Dear Editor-in-Chief,

Here in the U.S., and across the globe, humans are practicing "social distancing" to protect themselves and others from the effects of the COVID-19 pandemic (CNN, 2020). However, social distancing has brought adverse side effects such as social isolation. Particularly, older adults are more vulnerable to this pandemic because they are experiencing extreme loss of physical, social, and psychological interaction, which is essential for their health and well-being, as well as they are at higher risk of morbidity and mortality from COVID-19 (Santini et al., 2020). To make matters worse, older adults are witnessing family members suffer due to job loss and financial difficulties, which may increase the risk of mental health concerns. Fear and anxiety, stress and depression may result in maladaptive coping mechanisms where turning to alcohol, tobacco, or other drugs while staying at home becomes habitual (Centers for Disease Control and Prevention [CDC], 2020b). During this time, the direct impact and secondary consequences of COVID-19 disproportionately impacts older adults marginalized by sexual orientation, racial, economic inequalities, and/or disability.

LGBTQA+ older adults

There are more than 3 million LGBTQA+ (LGBT) older adults aged 55 and older living in the United States (SAGE, 2020a). They frequently experience discrimination from health care providers and barriers to health care services, increasing health disparities (Human Rights Watch, 2018). In addition, LGBT-related discrimination has put them at a higher risk of poverty and poor health outcomes such as depression (Greenesmith, 2017). Nearly 40% of LGBT older adults report being susceptible to loneliness as they were rejected by family or close friends because of gender identity or sexual orientation (Adams & Renteria, 2019). To this end, COVID-19 may exacerbate social isolation among this at-risk population.

Racial and ethnic minority older adults

Current statistics report that nearly 23% of the total population of older adults aged 65 and above are part of a racial and ethnic minority group (Administration for Community Living [ACL], 2018). Across races, Black and Hispanic individuals are overrepresented in reported statistics and are dying at a rate faster than compared to Whites from COVID-19 (Centers for Disease Control and Prevention [CDC], 2020a). Asians, and those who appear to be of Asian descent, are experiencing substantial incidents of bias, xenophobia, violence, and racism. This discrimination may result in a lack of health care access and treatment. On top of this, many ethnic and racial minorities are uninsured (Sohn, 2017) and lack primary health care providers (Hostetter & Klien, 2018), thus impacting care within the larger health care delivery system which is critical during this pandemic.

Low socioeconomic status

Likewise, economic stability is a major concern among older adults. Older adults of low socioeconomic status may be denied housing, can be evicted, or may lose federal rental assistance if found to be exposed to or test positive for COVID-19 (SAGE, 2020a). Roughly 15% of older adults live below the official poverty threshold (American Psychological Association [APA], n.d.). To counteract the rising costs of living and incidence of poverty, many older adults are working later in life (Cahill et al., 2013). Remaining in the workforce is especially dangerous during this pandemic placing this population at a heightened risk for exposure and contraction of COVID-19.

Older adults with disabilities

Among older adults with disabilities, basic needs of Activities of Daily Living (ADLs) such as assistance with bathing, basic home cleaning, and dementia supports may be unmet. A fear of going to medical facilities can prevent older adults from receiving needed physical, occupational, or speech therapy. Otherwise, serious illnesses unrelated to COVID-19 may be minimized or untreated (Berian et al., 2018). Despite many efforts for delivering services remotely such as telehealth, phone calls, or any other virtual communication during the pandemic outbreak, online technologies might be limited due to difficulties in access to digital resources (Armitagea & Nellumsa, 2020; Santini et al., 2020). For some, hearing loss, cognitive impairment, and unfamiliarity with new technology are additional barriers to services.

The disproportionate impact of COVID-19 on marginalized older adult is part of larger social justice issues. Social workers are in a unique position to address the impact of COVID-19 on vulnerable populations, promoting disease prevention efforts and helping address mental health issues through positive coping and cognitive behavioral therapies (Käll et al., 2020; National Association of Social Workers [NASW], 2020). Although many social workers may not conduct in-home visits during this time, or these practices may be limited, it is still imperative that we address the issues, including social isolation, loneliness, disparities in service delivery, and social exclusion through virtual engagement, service enrollment, and understanding diversity in aging.

Virtual engagement

Social workers ought to inquire about unmet social or functional needs with engaging with older adults through virtual service delivery. Leveraging social network platforms such as Twitter and Facebook to share messages and supportive resources can assist in engagement and connection with others. Establishing virtual friendly-visiting programs and engaging volunteers to make daily phone calls to older adults may reduce consequences of social isolation.

Service enrollment

Linking vulnerable older adults to services and supports is especially important during a pandemic crisis. Nutrition services authorized under Title III-C of the Older Americans Act (S. 192, 2015) are designed to promote the general health and well-being of older adults. Services are intended to reduce hunger, food insecurity and malnutrition, promote socialization, and delay the onset of adverse health conditions with special focus on low-income older adults, minority older adults, those in rural communities, with limited English proficiency, and seniors at risk of institutional care.

Understanding of diversity in aging

As America's population is becoming more diverse, how society and service agencies prepare for the increasing needs of diverse older adults is a big concern in gerontological social work (Steinman et al., 2020). Particularly, in the context of coping with stress, we need to understand that cultural groups react differently to stressful situations like COVID-19. Accordingly, it is imperative to identify coping strategies of older adults taking into consideration their cultural background, as psychological well-being may be affected by adaptive or maladaptive coping strategies (SAGE, 2020b).

Sincerely,

HeeSoon Lee and Vivian J. Miller

http://orcid.org/0000-0003-2030-862X

References

Adams, M., & Renteria, J. (2019). *LGBT older adults and immigrant care workers: What do they have in common?* American Society on Aging. https://www.asaging.org/blog/lgbt-older-adults-and-immigrant-care-workers-what-do-they-have-common

Administration for Community Living [ACL]. (2018). *2018 profile of older Americans.* https://acl.gov/sites/default/files/Aging%20and%20Disability%20in%20America/2018OlderAmericansProfile.pdf

American Psychological Association [APA]. (n.d.). *Fact sheet: Age and socioeconomic status.* https://www.apa.org/pi/ses/resources/publications/age

Armitagea, R., & Nellumsa, L. B. (2020). COVID-19 and the consequences of isolating the elderly. *Lancet Public Health, 5*(5), e256. https://doi.org/10.1016/S2468-2667(20)30061-X

Berian, J. R., Rosenthal, R. A., Baker, T. L., Coleman, J., Finlayson, E., Katlic, M. R., Lagoo-Deenadayalan, S. A., Tang, V. L., Robinson, T. N., Ko, C. Y., & Russell, M. M. (2018). Hospital standards to promote optimal surgical care of the older adult: A report from the coalition for quality in geriatric surgery. *Annals of Surgery, 267*(2), 280–290. https://doi.org/10.1097/SLA.0000000000002185

Cahill, K. E., Giandrea, M. D., & Quinn, J. F. (2013). Bridge employment. In M. Wang (Ed.), *Oxford library of psychology. The Oxford handbook of retirement* (pp. 293–310). Oxford University Press.

Centers for Disease Control and Prevention [CDC]. (2020a). *COVID-19 in racial and ethnic minority groups.* https://www.cdc.gov/coronavirus/2019-ncov/need-extra-precautions/racial-ethnic-minorities.html

Centers for Disease Control and Prevention [CDC]. (2020b). *Older adults.* https://www.cdc.gov/coronavirus/2019-ncov/need-extra-precautions/older-adults.html

CNN (2020). *These states have implemented stay-at-home orders. Here's what that means for you.* https://www.cnn.com/2020/03/23/us/coronavirus-which-states-stay-at-home-order-trnd/index.html

Greenesmith, H. (2017). *Aging as LGBT: Two stories.* Justice in Aging. https://www.justiceinaging.org/aging-as-lgbt/

Hostetter, M., & Klien, S. (2018). *In focus: Reducing racial disparities in health care by confronting racism.* The Commonwealth Fund. https://www.commonwealthfund.org/publications/newsletter-article/2018/sep/focus-reducing-racial-disparities-health-care-confronting

Human Rights Watch. (2018). *You don't want second best.* https://www.hrw.org/report/2018/07/23/you-dont-want-second-best/anti-lgbt-discrimination-us-health-care

Käll, A., Jägholm, S., Hesse, H., Andersson, F., Mathaldi, A., Norkvist, B. T., Shafran, R., & Andersson, G. (2020). Internet-based cognitive behavior therapy for loneliness: A pilot randomized controlled trial. *Behavior Therapy, 51*(1), 54–68. https://doi.org/10.1016/j.beth.2019.05.001

National Association of Social Workers [NASW]. (2020). *COVID resources and updates for social workers.* https://www.naswtx.org/news/492773/COVID-19-Resources–Updates-for-Social-Workers.htm

Older Americans Act Reauthorization Act of 2015, S. 192, 114th Cong. (2015). Congress.gov. https://www.congress.gov

SAGE (2020a). *Advocacy and services for LGBT elders.* https://www.diverseelders.org/issue/sage/

SAGE and Human Rights Campaign Foundation (2020b). https://dallasvoice.com/national-lgbt-health-organizations-warn-about-risks-of-covid-19-for-lgbtq-population/

Santini, Z., Jose, P., Cornwell, E., Koyanagi, A., Nielsen, L., Hinrichsen, C., Meilstrup, C., Madsen, K. R., & Koushede, V. (2020). Social disconnectedness, perceived isolation, and symptoms of depression and anxiety among older Americans (NSHAP): A longitudinal mediation analysis. *Lancet Public Health*, *5*(1), e62–e70. https://doi.org/10.1016/S2468-2667(19)30230-0

Sohn, H. (2017). Racial and ethnic disparities in health insurance coverage: Dynamics of gaining and losing coverage over the life-course. *Population Research and Policy Review*, *36*(2), 181–201. https://doi.org/10.1007/s11113-016-9416-y

Steinman, M. A., Perry, L., & Perissinotto, C. M. (2020). Meeting the care needs of older adults isolated at home during the COVID-19 pandemic. *JAMA Internal Medicine*. https://doi.org/10.1001/jamainternmed.2020.1661

Social Workers Must Address Intersecting Vulnerabilities among Noninstitutionalized, Black, Latinx, and Older Adults of Color during the COVID-19 Pandemic

Megan T. Ebor ⓘ, Tamra B. Loeb, and Laura Trejo

ABSTRACT

Scant attention has been paid to intersecting vulnerabilities experienced by Black, Latinx, and older adults of color (BLOAC) that increase COVID-19 related risks. Structural inequities have resulted in disproportionate rates of chronic conditions and limited access to care. Media coverage, focused on COVID-19 mortality among institutionalized older adults (OA), has overlooked community-dwelling OA, leaving their unique risks unaddressed in research and intervention efforts. Key vulnerabilities impacting noninstitutionalized BLOAC exacerbating adverse health outcomes during COVID-19 are discussed, and recommendations are given for gerontological social work (GSW) education, training, and practice to meet the needs of BLOAC during the COVID-19 pandemic.

Increasing evidence indicates that health disparities, in addition to age and underlying chronic medical conditions (e.g., diabetes, heart, and lung disease), increase COIVD-19 related risks among Black, Latinx, and Older Adults of Color (BLOAC) due to long standing structural inequities in the United States (Centers for Disease Control, 2020a). These risks tend to be discussed individually; little attention is paid to how vulnerabilities intersect to heighten risks for serious COIVD-19 related illness and death (Centers for Disease Control, 2020b). Media coverage of older adults (OAs) highlight COVID-mortality rates in nursing homes; however, the vast majority of OAs in the U.S. are community dwelling (Howley, 2019); thus, noninstitutionalized BLOAC needs have not received adequate attention. Social workers are uniquely positioned to bring visibility to this population and address their distinctive COVID-19 vulnerabilities.

Back, Latinx and older adults of color are a rapidly growing population in the U.S. (Administration for Community Living, 2018), experiencing disproportionately high rates of preventable disease, disability, and death due to differences in sociodemographic conditions that pose barriers to prevention, health and insurance access, and treatment efforts (Centers for Disease Control, 2020a; Williams, 2007). Approximately 80% of COVID-related mortalities in the U.S. are among adults 65 years and older (Centers for Disease Control, 2020b; Nania, 2020). Physical distancing mandates will likely exacerbate long standing mental and physical health disparities among community-dwelling BLOAC (Novacek et al., 2020). Research has yet to identify the best way to help this population adapt to this pandemic. Social work clinicians and researchers, at the forefront of programmatic innovation, dissemination of COVID-19 related information, and linkages to care during these unprecedented times, are uniquely qualified to address the needs of BLOAC. To do so, SWs must draw upon their knowledge base that acknowledges differential access to resources (Ingrao, 2015). While strides have been made to cultivate interest in geriatric social work (GSW), this subfield lacks visibility (Sanders et al., 2017), yet is certain to face increased demand to address the needs of BLOAC, particularly surrounding COVID-19. The following recommendations for SW clinicians and training programs are proposed:

(1) Prioritize GSW educational and training opportunities. Gerontological content should be infused throughout SW curricula, increasing exposure to the field of GSW, awareness of the diverse needs of OA to mitigate health disparities among BLOAC, and providing GSW training opportunities in community settings to prepare SWs to work to combat adverse COIVD-19 related outcomes among BLOAC.

(2) Provide services that decrease social isolation and link clients with needed services via telehealth platforms. Social services and social clubs should adapt existing services to incorporate virtual programming. Villages and CBOs can be used to maintain social connectedness. Over 40% of OAs own smartphones and 67% have internet access; yet, only 25% feel confident accessing information online (Anderson & Perrin, 2017). Social workers can connect OAs to resources that assist with tech-utilization and promote telephone reassurance programs where trained volunteers provide calls serving as "well-checks" and provide socializing opportunities (Slootmaker, 2020).

(3) Assessments should include healthy coping opportunities to mitigate COVID-19 related stress, including religion, faith, and/or spirituality histories (significant in over 90% of OA); culturally humble practice recognizes these as resources that can provide vitality, wellbeing and optimism during crises (Kaplan & Berkman, 2019; Malone & Dadswell, 2018). Practitioners can initiate partnerships with faith organizations to creatively maintain spiritual connections by providing trusted testing spaces for BLOAC, food distribution, modified engagement via telephone prayer lines, and virtual support groups.

COVID-19 presents complex concerns for BLOAC. A focus on GSW is needed in the field. Linking BLOAC to services using telehealth to maintain social connectedness, using modified interactions via religiosity and/or spirituality are suggested as interventions to decrease risks and promote better health management during this pandemic.

Funding

This work was supported by the National Heart, Lung, and Blood Institute [3U01HL 142109-02W1].

ORCID

Megan T. Ebor ⓘ http://orcid.org/0000-0001-8796-634X

References

Administration for Community Living. (2018). *Profile of older Americans*. United States Department of Health and Human Services. https://acl.gov/sites/default/files/Aging%20and%20Disability%20in%20America/2018OlderAmericansProfile.pdf

Anderson, M., & Perrin, A. (2017). *Tech adoption climbs among older adults*. Pew research center. Internet and technology. Retrieved from https://www.pewresearch.org/internet/2017/05/17/tech-adoption-climbs-among-older-adults/

Centers for Disease Control and Prevention (2020a). *COVID-19 guidance for older adults*. https://www.cdc.gov/aging/covid19-guidance.html

Centers for Disease Control and Prevention (2020b). Older Adults. *Coronavirus Disease 2019 (COVID-19)*. https://www.cdc.gov/coronavirus/2019-ncov/need-extra-precautions/older-adults.html

Howley, E. K. (2019, October). Nursing home facts and statistics. U.S. News. Retrieved from https://health.usnews.com/health-news/best-nursing-homes/articles/nursing-home-facts-andstatistics

Ingrao, C. (2015). Gerontological social work: Meeting the needs of an aging population. Social Work at Simmons. Retrieved from https://socialwork.simmons.edu/gerontological-social-work-meeting-needs-aging-population/

Kaplan, D. B., & Berkman, B. J., (2019). *Religion and spirituality in older adults*. Merck Manual Professional version. Merck Sharp & Dohme Corp. Retrieved from https://www.merckmanuals.com/professional/geriatrics/social-issues-in-older-adults/religion-and-spirituality-in-older-adults

Malone, J., & Dadswell, A. (2018). The role of religion, spirituality and/or belief in positive ageing for older adults. *Geriatrics (Basel, Switzerland)*, *3*(2), 28. doi:10.3390/geriatrics3020028.

Nania, R. (2020). *Blacks, hispanics hit harder by the Coronavirus, early U.S. data show*. *American Association of Retired Persons (AARP)*. https://www.aarp.org/health/conditions-treatments/info-2020/minority-communities-covid-19.html

Novacek, D. M., Hampton-Anderson, J. N., Ebor, M. T., Loeb, T. B., & Wyatt, G. E. (2020). Mental health ramifications of the COVID-19 pandemic for Black Americans: Clinical and research recommendations. *Psychological Trauma: Theory, Research, Practice, and Policy*. Advance online publication. http://dx.doi.org/10.1037/tra0000796

Sanders, S., Anderson, K. A., Berg-Weger, M., Kaplan, D., & Schroepfer, T. (2017). Association for Gerontology Education in Social Work (AGESW): Key initiatives and directions. *Journal of Gerontological Social Work, 60*(5), 330–334. https://doi.org/10.1080/01634372.2017.1363596

Slootmaker, E., (2020, May). Friendly reassurance calls help Michigan elders fight isolation during pandemic. Second Wave. Retrieved from https://www.secondwavemedia.com/features/friendlyreassurance05142020.aspx

Williams, M. (2007). Invisible, unequal, and forgotten: health disparities in the Elderly. Notre Dame journal of law. *Ethics & Public Policy, 21*(2), 441–478.

Expanding Bilingual Social Workers for the East Asian Older Adults beyond the "COVID-19 Racism"

Dear Editor,

On March 11, 2020, the World Health Organization announced that the outbreak of COVID-19 was a public health emergency of international concern after thousands of cases of the virus had been confirmed throughout the world. As the virus continued to spread, the world began to concentrate on how to stop it. In spite of the global effort to stop the virus, however, unforeseen racial issues have emerged among the East Asian community, and they have found themselves targeted as carriers of the virus and have been subjected to random acts of violence. Particularly vulnerable to this kind of racism are the East Asian older adults who are already facing social issues like inadequate health and social services due to their cultural and linguistic barriers in the U.S (Na et al., 2016; Yoo et al., 2015). Existing issues experienced by East Asian older adults are exacerbated by racism related to COVID-19.

In 2014, the older Asian American population was 1.9 million, and it is projected to grow to 8.5 million by 2060. Even with this projection, Asian health and social needs in the U.S. can be easily overlooked (Museus & Iftikar, 2014). Poverty rates for adults aged 65 and older in 2015 are nine percent, while those of Asian adults are close to eighteen percent according to the 2015 American Community Survey one-year estimate. Asian older adults, especially those who are foreign-born, receive on average, lower Social Security benefits than their peers (Tran, 2017). Asian American older adults are also the most vulnerable to mental health issues such as depression and suicide. (Na et al., 2016; Yoo et al., 2015). Their mental health service utilization is the lowest out of all older adults' groups due to a lack of culturally and linguistically sensitive services (Yang et al., 2019). The Asian immigrant population has the highest language barrier, with thirty-five percent speaking English "less than very well" (United States Census Bureau, 2019). According to the latest report on East Asian older adults in New York (Center for an Urban Future, 2013), their limited English proficiency (LEP) rates are much higher than any other group: Chinese older adults (92%) and Korean older adults (94%). Due to all these factors, Asian older adults are highly likely to move to Asian American cultural hubs in large metropolitan cities for more social engagement and community support. Unfortunately, these metropolitan cultural hubs also incur higher housing and living costs, which negatively affect older adults in the long term (Tran, 2017).

To further complicate matters, COVID racism is spreading fast. The incorrect reference to COVID-19 virus as the "Chinese virus," and "Wuhan virus" has solidified misconceptions and led to a violent racial backlash against the East Asian population. A Chinese woman was attacked for wearing a mask in New York City while a 16-year-old Asian American student was physically assaulted in Los Angeles (Ao, 2020). In Canada, a 92-year-old Asian man with dementia was attacked by a white man who shouted racial slurs about COVID-19 (Young, May 13, 2020). Similar racial attacks have happened all over the world. There is a strong link between racial discrimination and anxiety and depression among diverse racial groups. Mental health professionals have already raised concerns about the impact of COVID racism against East Asians, especially its effects on the older adults' population (Ao, 2020).

Yet, no intervention has been studied or developed for East Asian older adults with LEP except for bilingual assistance from the community. Bilingual assistance in community-based ethnic organizations is heavily dependent upon volunteers due to a lack of bilingual social workers (Weng, 2014). However, bilingual volunteers cannot provide social and mental health services and interventions as social workers do (Weng, 2014). There is hardly any research or information on Asian bilingual social workers and their service delivery status in the fields. Reports from the Council on Social Work Education (CSWE) only indicate that less than 3% of MSW and BSW graduates were of Asian descendent between 2015 and 2018 (Council on Social Work Education, 2016, 2018, 2019).

Considering East Asian older adults are in dire need of both social and mental health services in the face of COVID-19 and COVID racism, Asian bilingual social workers are needed now more than ever. These social workers can communicate with them, help them, and advocate for them with professional knowledge and ethical obligation to promote their wellbeing. So far, no attention has been made to promote bilingual social workers from any reasonable parties such as community-based organizations or social work program institutions. As an East Asian bilingual social worker who has been providing services to older adults in the one of the metropolitan cities in the U.S., I would like to encourage these responsible parties to collaborate to build future social workers. By supporting bilingual volunteers in the community to attend social work programs, the community will gain more bilingual social workers in the Asian community when social work professionals are more diverse. In this way, East Asian older adults can take active and affirmative action on their existing issues and COVID racism with help from Asian bilingual social workers.

Sangeun Lee

ⓘ http://orcid.org/0000-0002-2062-2523

References

Ao, B. (2020, April 22). Asian Americans already face a mental health crisis. Coronavirus racism could make it worse. *The Philadelphia Inquirer*. https://www.inquirer.com/health/coronavirus/coronavirus-racism-asian-americans-mental-health-20200422.html

Center for an Urban Future. (2013, July). The new face of New York's seniors, pp. 1-56. Retrieved from https://nycfuture.org/pdf/The-New-Face-of-New-Yorks-Seniors.pdf

Council on Social Work Education. (2016). *CSWE annual report 20152016*.https://www.cswe.org/getattachment/About-CSWE/Annual-Reports/CSWE-Annual-Reports/cswe_2015-2016AnnualReport_web.pdf.aspx

Council on Social Work Education. (2018). *CSWE annual report 20162017*.https://cswe.org/getattachment/About-CSWE/Annual-Reports/CSWE-Annual-Reports/CSWE-Annual-Report-2017.pdf.aspx

Council on Social Work Education. (2019). *CSWE annual report 2018*. https://cswe.org/getattachment/Research-Statistics/Annual-Program-Study/2018-Statistics-on-Social-Work-Education-in-the-United-States.pdf.aspx

Museus, S. D., & Iftikar, J. (2014). Asian Critical Theory (AsianCrit). In M. Y. Danico & J. G. Golsom (Eds.), *Asian American society*. Thousand Oaks, CA: Sage Publications and Association for Asian American Studies. http://works.bepress.com/samuel_museus/91/.

Na, S., Ryder, A. G., & Kirmayer, K. J. (2016, September 5). Toward a culturally responsive model of mental health literacy: Facilitating help-seeking among East Asian immigrants to north America. *Community Psychology, 58*, 211–225. https://doi-org.proxy.brynmawr.edu/10.1002/ajcp.12085

Tran, V. (2017, May 30). Asian American seniors are often left out of the national conversation on poverty. *The Urban Institute 58*, 211–225. https://www.urban.org/urban-wire/asian-american-seniors-are-often-left-out-national-conversation-poverty

United States Census Bureau. (2019, January 24). *2020 census barriers, attitudes, and motivators study survey report*. U.S. Department of Commerce. https://www2.census.gov/programs-surveys/decennial/2020/program-management/final-analysis-reports/2020-report-cbams-study-survey.pdf

Weng, S. S. (2014). Founding of ethnic programs and agencies for Asian Americans: An exploration of strategies & challenges. *Human Service Organizations: Management, Leadership & Governance, 38*(1), 55–73. https://doi.org/10.1080/03643107.2013.853010

World Health Organizations. (2020, April 14). *COVID 19 strategy update*. https://www.who.int/docs/default-source/coronaviruse/covid-strategy-update-14april2020.pdf?sfvrsn=29da3ba0_19

World Health Organizations, Bulletin of the World Health Organization. (2020). *Novel coronavirus (COVID-19)*. https://www.who.int/emergencies/diseases/novel-coronavirus-2019

Yang, K. G., Rodgers, Caryn R. R.., Lee, E.. Lê Cook, E. B.A., & Lê Cook, B. (2019, October 2). Disparities in Mental Health Care Utilization and Perceived Need Among Asian Americans: 2012–2016. Psychiatric Services. Retrieved from https://ps.psychiatryonline.org/doi/full/10.1176/appi.ps.201900126 1 71 21-27 doi:10.1176/appi.ps.201900126

Yoo, G. J., Musselman, E., Lee, Y., & Yee-Melichar, D. (2015). Addressing health disparities among older Asian Americans: Data and diversity. *ASA's Quarterly Journal, Generations 38* (4), 74-81. https://www.asaging.org/blog/addressing-health-disparities-among-older-asian-americans-data-and-diversity.

Young, I. (2020, May 13). Coronavirus: Asian women in Canada are abused, punched and spat on. Is it racist maskaphobia? *The Coronavirus Pandemic*. The South China Morning Post. Retrieved from https://www.scmp.com/news/world/united-states-canada/article/3084090/coronavirus-asian-women-canada-are-abused-punched

Older Latinx Immigrants and Covid-19: A Call to Action

Dear Editor,

As the U.S. ages it will also become more ethnoracially diverse. While the share of non-Latinx white elders is expected to drop from 78% to 54% in the next few decades, the share of older Latinxs is projected to double, from 16% to 28%, during the same period (Mather et al., 2015). Three in four of these Latinx baby boomers were born in Latin America (Gassoumis et al., 2010).

There are a number of reasons to pay attention to the impact of Covid-19 on older Latinx immigrants. *First*, inequities exists concerning access to information related to the novel Coronavirus. While the World Health Organization and the Center for Disease Control and Prevention have issued Coronavirus guidelines in Spanish, it may be challenging for older immigrants who are not proficient in English to access this information because many do not rely on the internet as a primary source of information (Yoon et al., 2020). Low levels of formal education compounded by limited health literacy (Calvo, 2016) may exacerbate access to accurate information about the pandemic and its effects. Older immigrants, therefore, may find it challenging to understand safeguards aimed to prevent contagion, such as how to remain safe while taking public transportation. *Second*, older immigrants may face a higher risk of infection if they live in close quarters with family members who are frontline workers or because they are frontline workers themselves. The pandemic has brought attention through news media of a system of racial inequality that channels Latinxs to jobs that have been deemed essential under stay-at-home advisories issued by governors, yet face shortages of measures, like personal protective equipment, to mitigate the possibility of contagion. *Third*, Latinx immigrants as a group have worse health and fewer resources to respond to the pandemic than other groups of older adults. A history of lifelong disadvantage stemming from systemic discrimination results in disproportionate high rates of obesity, hypertension, diabetes and functional limitations in later life (Martinez & Baron, 2020). These challenges are compounded by restricted opportunities to tap into the safety net. Some immigrants are undocumented and thus barred from benefits. Others do not have a work history in the United States; or if they do have, it is not long enough to qualify for services (Jacqueline L. Angel & Berlinger, 2018). Even for the entitled, the safety net is not as widely cast as it is for other American seniors. Unlike many older adults with employer-sponsored retirement plans, Latinx immigrants tend to rely exclusively on Social Security and Supplemental Security Income (SSI) as their main sources of income late in life (Ronald J. Angel & Angel, 2015). *Fourth*, systemic inequities on access to long-term care and community-based services place older Latinxs at high risk of experiencing lack of health care, food insecurity and economic hardship (Sadarangani & Murali, 2018). Elders may not know how to navigate the system of social protection, may be unaware of services offered in the community, such as food banks and food deliveries for older adults, or believe that they are ineligible for services, or that the services are for purchase rather than for free. *Fifth*, the current wide-spread anti-immigrant rhetoric reflected in actions like the Public Charge rule has made immigrants reluctant to seek health care or to apply for age-related benefits for fear of immigration-related repercussions for themselves and for their families (Ayón et al., 2020). The Public Charge rule establishes that immigrants may be denied permanent residency in the US if they are deemed dependent on public benefits including health care, nutrition, or housing (Bernstein et al., 2020). Older Latinx immigrants, as a result, may avoid getting tested for the coronavirus or may forego healthcare altogether because they are afraid of sharing personal information.

Understanding how these older immigrants are faring during the pandemic and its aftermath will help advocates, providers of services and policy makers to design services tailored to this population. This is important for two related reasons. *First*, because there is a lack of alternative frameworks for understanding elder services within Latinx populations. The assumption that older Latinxs prefer to rely on the family rather that in formal services may increase inequalities by preventing providers of services, advocates and policy makers from pursuing systemic changes that increase the access to services for older Latinx immigrants. It also prevents the creating of culturally-congruent resources to be deployed when working with this community. *Second*, because there is a lack of involvement of people most affected by the pandemic in problem-solving strategies that can be implemented systemically. We will be dealing with how to respond to the COVID-19 for months to come. Hence, understanding, for instance, the most effective way to create and distribute information among older Latinxs from their own perspective may help decrease inequities in access to future therapeutic treatments for Covid-19. In the same fashion, examining how the pandemic has eroded the safety nets of older Latinxs, including family supports and social relationships, and proposing actions that are led by the community itself will help providers of services and policy makers to design responses tailored to meet the needs of this population.

Rocío Calvo

ⓘ http://orcid.org/0000-0002-6303-9215

Conflicts of interest

The author has no conflicts of interest to declare.

Funding

This research was funded by Russell Sage Foundation [Grant #:1902-11556].

References

Angel, J. L., & Berlinger, N. (2018). The Trump administration's assault on health and social programs: Potential consequences for older Hispanics. *Journal of Aging and Social Policy, 30* (3–4), 300–315. https://doi.org/10.1080/08959420.2018.1462678

Angel, R. J., & Angel, J. L. (2015). *Latinos in an aging world: Social, psychological, and economic perspectives.* Routledge.

Ayón, C., Ramos Santiago, J., & López Torres, A. S. (2020). Latinx undocumented older adults, health needs and access to healthcare. *Journal of Immigrants and Minority Health.* https://doi.org/10.1007/s10903-019-00966-7

Bernstein, H., Gonzalez, D., Karpman, M., & Zuckerman, S. (2020). *Amid confusion over the public charge rule, immigrant families continued avoiding public benefits in 2019.* Urban Institute. Available at https://www.urban.org/research/publication/amid-confusion-overpublic-charge-rule-immigrant-families-continued-avoiding-public-benefits-2019

Calvo, R. (2016). Health literacy and quality of care among Latino immigrants. *Health & Social Work, 41*(1), e44–e51. https://doi.org/10.1093/hsw/hlv076

Gassoumis, Z. D., Wilber, K. H., Baker, L. A., & Torres-Gil, F. M. (2010). Who are the latino baby boomers? Demographic and economic characteristics of a hidden population. *Journal of Aging & Social Policy, 22*(1), 53–68. https://doi.org/10.1080/08959420903408452

Martinez, I. L., & Baron, A. (2020). Aging and health in the Latinx population in the USA: changing demographics, social vulnerabilities, and the aim of quality of life. In A. Martínez & S. Rhodes (Eds.), *New and emerging issues in Latinx health* (pp. 145–168). Springer.

Mather, M., Jacobsen, L. A., & Pollard, K. M. (2015). Population Bulletin. *Population Reference Bureau, 70*(2). https://assets.prb.org/pdf16/aging-us-population-bulletin.pdf

Sadarangani, T. R., & Murali, K. P. (2018). Service use, participation, experiences, and outcomes among older adult immigrants in American adult day service centers: An integrative review of the literature. *Research in Gerontological Nursing, 11*(6), 317–328. https://doi.org/10.3928/19404921-20180629-01

Yoon, H., Jang, Y., Waughan, P. W., & Garcia, M. (2020). Older adults' internet use for health information: Digital divide by race/ethnicity and socioeconomic status. *Journal of Applied Gerontology, 39*(1), 105–110. https://doi.org/10.1177/0733464818770772

Social Work Response Needed to the Challenge of COVID-19 for Aging People with Intellectual and Developmental Disabilties

Dear Editor,

The COVID-19 pandemic affects all of us, but consequences are more serious for those who are older or have chronic conditions and immune disorders. Places where numbers of people are living together, such as in nursing homes, have also proven to be particularly vulnerable. People with intellectual and developmental disabilities (I/DD) frequently present with the same risk factors but are largely forgotten in the care, response, and policy discussion.

Reports in New York are that people with I/DD have infections and death rates higher than the general population (Hakim, 2020). Although there is no evidence yet that having an I/DD, itself is a risk factor for COVID-19, well-documented health inequities (McCallion et al., 2017) for people with I/DD as they age are compounding risks:

- they have higher levels than others of multi-morbidity including heart and respiratory diseases and immune disorders;
- there are barriers they experience in accessing health care particularly as a group who have difficulty in describing symptoms; and
- historic stigma and views that their lives are less valuable pose additional risk, if decisions occur about who receives care when resources are scarce.

Many individuals with I/DD live with multiple people, and some do not understand the concept of keeping distance. Others have difficulty in reporting their symptoms, do not understand instructions for self-care, and experience imposed isolation and quarantining as punishing and bewildering. The places where people with I/DD live are not set up to support isolation spaces and, as was also noted by Hakim (2020), they have not been a priority for personal protective equipment (PPE) distribution. Finally, although the response of many service providers has been to "lock down" these settings with no visitors and no trips outside the home, there has necessarily been daily entry and exit of staff who themselves are largely untested, rarely have PPE and who may feel obligated to come to work even if unwell. The service system was unprepared for COVID-19 at multiple levels and now needs to think about what will be different the next time. It needs the social workers in the system to not simply insist on change but to help build a pandemic/natural disaster responsive infrastructure.

When a person with I/DD is living at home, we have learned we need to be concerned about the risks for other family members, as well, particularly if the caregivers themselves are older and have their own chronic conditions. Future planning among persons with I/DD has been mostly focused upon transitions out of the family homes. Social workers, working in care management roles, must give equal attention to back-up plans, when caregivers becomes ill, and to advanced care planning for both the caregiver and the person with I/DD.

Individuals with I/DD regardless of where they live are falling through the cracks as frequently they are not a priority for testing or care–not because healthcare workers are uncaring, but because, as has been demonstrated in many communities our systems and staff are overwhelmed. Social work needs to be at the forefront of creating disability-friendly pathways to testing and care.

As rates of infection and of mortality appear to decline there is still a concern that there may be new "spikes" of infection, and potentially new waves of reoccurrence. For those with I/DD, service providers must radically respond by thinking about the person themselves, the individuals they live with, and protective strategies for the home. Training is needed for extra vigilance for symptoms for family members and staff working in settings with people who have I/DD. Procedures and strategies are needed for taking seriously any symptoms observed, rather than attributing such symptoms to disability.

Attention should be geared to promoting activities that encourage staying home, handwashing, and keeping physical distance. In isolation or quarantine, we all benefit from physical activity – one can find videos and come up with games, songs, and stories that include chair exercises or in-home physical activity. These activities also work for those who are caring for someone with I/DD. Pandemics/natural disasters call upon us all to be our most creative in providing and managing these activities.

Restricting our activities and staying in place will make many of us feel increasingly isolated. For people with I/DD, who often have smaller social groups and have fewer opportunities to find virtual alternatives, this loss of key connections will be felt even more. Family and staff can help here, too. Social work attention is needed to planning and implementing alternative forms of contacts, including virtual so that they can be inclusive, anticipated, and enjoyed by those with disabilities, rather than missed.

Perhaps most challenging is to have honest conversations about care when persons with I/DD experience serious and life-threatening symptoms. There has rightly been concern about the potential that in overwhelming situations such as in pandemics, care may be rationed and the criteria used may disadvantage people with disabilities. Social workers are already advocating to ensure that disability is not a criterion for exclusion (AASWSW, 2020). Decisions on whether to place people with I/DD in hospital, often unaccompanied, when infected, and/or to place them on ventilators in their last days also have their controversies. Social workers should be advocates that such decisions be guided by advanced care planning in which the persons with I/DD themselves have participated if possible.

Going forward, from this experience with a pandemic there are as well as practice and policy concerns, research needs for social work to address. These include documenting among people with I/DD the incidence and experience of COVID-19, successes and failures in offering support, and development and testing of interventions. The inclusion of people with I/DD and family members as co-researchers should be supported.

Philip McCallion

✉ philip.mccallion@temple.edu

References

AASWSW. (2020). *Policy of the American Academy of Social Work and Social Welfare (AASWSW) on the right of all Americans to potential life saving vaccinations and care.*

Hakim, D. (2020, April 9). *'It's Hit Our Front Door': Homes for the Disabled See a Surge of Covid-19.* New York Times. https://www.nytimes.com/2020/04/08/nyregion/coronavirus-disabilities-group-homes.html

McCallion, P., Jokinen, N., & Janicki, M. P. (2017). Aging. In A comprehensive guide to intellectual and developmental disabilities, M.I. Wehmeyer, Brown, M., Percey, S. K., & Fung, M. (Eds), *Pp. 639-654.* MD: Paul Brookes Press: Baltimore.

Unraveling the Invisible but Harmful Impact of COVID-19 on Deaf Older Adults and Older Adults with Hearing Loss

Dear Editor-in-Chief,

As the unpredictable but devastating impact of the COVID-19 pandemic continues, health disparities among population groups become increasingly wider. The Centers for Disease Control and Prevention (CDC) has identified older adults as particularly vulnerable to COVID-19; in fact, they account for the largest proportion (about 80%) of deaths caused by the virus (CDC, 2020). Researchers have looked for ways to prevent and treat COVID-19 in older adults; however, when developing innovative and effective interventions to reduce adverse COVID-19 outcomes, older adults who experience daily communication difficulties have not been adequately considered. This population consists of two groups based on their main communication mode: (a) Deaf older adults (DOA), who primarily use American Sign Language (ASL) and (b) older adults with hearing loss (OAHL), including Hard of Hearing older adults and older adults with age-related hearing loss (HL; presbycusis), who primarily use spoken English or other spoken languages.

Although statistics for the number of DOA and OAHL affected by COVID-19 are currently unavailable, these populations could be more vulnerable than hearing older adults. It is important for social workers to understand the unique challenges of these populations in order to develop interventions to combat adverse COVID-19 outcomes.

Low health literacy and knowledge about COVID-19

While hearing older adults can easily obtain health information via incidental learning through spoken language, DOA and OAHL have limited access to spoken language-focused family and social engagement (Lesch et al., 2019; Panzer et al., 2020). As a result, they are more likely to have inadequate health literacy (Kushalnagar & Kushalnagar, 2018; McKee et al., 2015; Wells et al., 2020). Recently, Kushalnagar (2020) discovered that Deaf and hard of hearing (D/HH) people who did not understand the importance of social distancing were less likely to perceive social distancing as an effective way to prevent the spread of COVID-19.

Inaccessible public information regarding COVID-19

Current public health information related to COVID-19 is largely disseminated via mass media or educational materials in written or spoken English (Murray, 2020; Panzer et al., 2020). Without access to information via ASL or subtitles, DOA and OAHL, especially those who might already have low health literacy, may struggle to access accurate information due to unfamiliar and complicated terminology. Drum et al. (2020) revealed that D/HH people found COVID-19 information via the Internet (34%), television (26%), and health-care providers (21%). DOA are more likely to use YouTube and other social media as health information sources (Kushalnagar & Kushalnagar, 2018). Despite the existence of some ASL-accessible health websites, DOA are still at greater risk for eHealth disparities because these information sources are not tailored to the needs of a heterogeneous D/HH community (Kushalnagar & Kushalnagar, 2018).

Higher prevalence of chronic diseases

Previous findings show that DOA and OAHL are more likely to have chronic conditions such as asthma, diabetes, high blood pressure, and stroke (McKee et al., 2018), all of which are risk factors for adverse COVID-19 outcomes (CDC, 2020). Furthermore, partly due to higher rates of chronic disease, these populations are already more likely to visit emergency rooms and hospitals or live in nursing homes and long-term care facilities (Frank, 2016; Genther et al., 2013), where the probability of contracting COVID-19 is high.

Unintended negative consequences of using face masks

Face masks, while being the most effective tool for preventing the spread of COVID-19 (CDC, 2020), have had unintended but significant health consequences for both DOA and OAHL. Masks create difficulty for DOA because they can hide visual cues such as facial expressions, which are necessary components of ASL communication. Face masks also compromise communication with OAHL by preventing lip reading and decreasing volume and accuracy (Perencevich et al., 2020; Tagupa, 2020). Masks can compromise acquisition of COVID-related information (i.e., preventive methods, test locations, coping with COVID-related risk factors), increasing their risk for adverse COVID-19 outcomes. Masks can also disrupt interpersonal communication in general (West et al., 2020), leading to social withdrawal and perhaps increasing social isolation, loneliness, and depression (Tagupa, 2020).

Inaccessible COVID-19 testing and healthcare services

DOA and OAHL traditionally have lower access to quality health care due to discordant communication with health-care providers, low knowledge among health-care providers about serving and communicating with DOA and OAHL, and the unavailability of reasonable accommodations (i.e., qualified ASL interpreters for doctors) (Blustein et al., 2018; Lesch et al., 2019; Panzer et al., 2020). The ubiquitous use of face masks among health-care providers may compromise COVID-19 testing and appropriate health care patients who are DOA or OAHL, in addition to ongoing difficulties in dealing with their chronic diseases (Recio-Barbero et al., 2020).

Given all of these factors, social workers should help develop alternative formats for disseminating COVID-related information and custom interventions that specifically target adverse COVID-19 outcomes in DOA and OAHL so that they are no longer so disproportionately at risk.

Junghyun Park

ⓘ http://orcid.org/0000-0001-7762-1807

References

Blustein, J., Weinstein, B. E., & Chodosh, J. (2018). Tackling hearing loss to improve the care of older adults. *British Medical Journal*, *360*, 1–4. https://doi.org/10.1136/bmj.k21

Centers for Disease Control and Prevention. (2020, June 19). *Coronavirus disease 2019 (COVID-19)*. Older Adults. https://www-cdc-gov.proxy.library.nyu.edu/coronavirus/2019-ncov/need-extra-precautions/older-adults.html

Drum, C. E., Oberg, A., Cooper, K., & Carlin, R. (2020). *COVID-19 & adults who are deaf or hard of hearing: Health and health care access online survey report*. American Association on Health and Disability.

Frank, A. K. (2016). Deaf seniors: Experiencing oppression. *Journal of the American Deafness & Rehabilitation Association*, *50*(2), 45–66.

Genther, D. J., Frick, K. D., Chen, D., Betz, J., & Lin, F. R. (2013). Association of hearing loss with hospitalization and burden of disease in older adults. *Jama*, *309*(22), 2322–2324. https://doi.org/10.1001/jama.2013.5912

Kushalnagar, P. (2020, June 27). *Part 1 findings from a survey of deaf Americans: COVID-19 awareness and risk perceptions*. 281560-1083163-raikfcquaxqncofqfm.stackpathdns.com/wp-content/uploads/2020/05/COVID-19-Deaf-Health-Report_2020.pdf

Kushalnagar, P., & Kushalnagar, R. (2018). Health-related information seeking among deaf adults: findings from the 2017 health information national trends survey in American sign language (HINTS-ASL). In *eHealth: Current evidence, promises, perils and future directions* (pp. 69–91). Emerald Publishing Limited.https://doi.org/10.1108/S2050-206020180000015008

Lesch, H., Burcher, K., Wharton, T., Chapple, R., & Chapple, K. (2019). Barriers to healthcare services and supports for signing deaf older adults. *Rehabilitation Psychology*, *64*(2), 237–244. https://doi.org/10.1037/rep0000252

McKee, M. M., Paasche-Orlow, M. K., Winters, P. C., Fiscella, K., Zazove, P., Sen, A., & Pearson, T. (2015). Assessing health literacy in deaf American sign language users. *Journal of Health Communication, 20*(2), 92–100. https://doi.org/10.1080/10810730.2015.1066468

McKee, M. M., Stransky, M. L., & Reichard, A. (2018). Hearing loss and associated medical conditions among individuals 65 years and older. *Disability and Health Journal, 11*(1), 122–125. https://doi.org/10.1016/j.dhjo.2017.05.007

Murray, J. J. (2020, June 19). Improving signed language and communication accessibility during COVID-19 pandemic. *The Hearing Journal.* https://journals.lww.com/thehearing journal/blog/OnlineFirst/pages/post.aspx?PostID=66

Panzer, K., Park, J., Pertz, L., & McKee, M. M. (2020). Teaming together to care for our deaf patients: Insights from the deaf health clinic. *Journal of the American Deafness & Rehabilitation Association, 53*(2), 60–77.

Perencevich, E. N., Diekema, D. J., & Edmond, M. B. (2020). Moving personal protective equipment into the community: Face shields and containment of COVID-19. *JAMA, 323* (22), 2252–2253. https://doi.org/10.1001/jama.2020.7477

Recio-Barbero, M., Sáenz-Herrero, M., & Segarra, R. (2020). Deafness and mental health: Clinical challenges during the COVID-19 pandemic. *Psychological Trauma: Theory, Research, Practice, and Policy, 12*(S1), S212–S213. https://doi.org/10.1037/tra0000729

Tagupa, H. (2020). Social isolation, loneliness, and hearing loss during COVID-19. *The Hearing Journal, 73*(5), 46–47. https://doi.org/10.1097/01.HJ.0000666456.65020.b9

Wells, T. S., Rush, S. R., Nickels, L. D., Wu, L., Bhattarai, G. R., & Yeh, C. S. (2020). Limited health literacy and hearing loss among older adults. *HLRP: Health Literacy Research and Practice, 4*(2), e129–e137. https://doi.org/10.3928/24748307-20200511-01

West, J. S., Franck, K. H., & Welling, D. B. (2020). Providing health care to patients with hearing loss during COVID–19 and physical distancing. *Laryngoscope Investigative Otolaryngology, 5*(3), 396–398. https://doi.org/10.1002/lio2.382

The Impact of COVID-19 on Older Adults Living with HIV: HIV Care and Psychosocial Effects

Dear Editor,

The COVID-19 pandemic continues to have a detrimental impact worldwide, and in the US. As of July 8, 2020, there were 11,892,382 cases worldwide with 545,485 deaths, and 3,016,515 cases in the US with 131,666 deaths (Johns Hopkins University, 2020). Groups that are at a higher risk to experience severe morbidity from COVID-19 include older adults and adults with underlying health conditions (diabetes, heart disease, lung disease, cancer, high blood pressure), and compromised immune systems. Indeed, COVID-19 and HIV have been considered a syndemic health challenge (Shiau et al., 2020). One group of people who are also among the vulnerable are older adults living with HIV. The effect of the COVID-19 and HIV syndemic may be more pronounced for this population (Shiau et al., 2020). Some older adults living with HIV undergo numerous challenges and facing another epidemic brings with it a host of additional challenges that are discussed below.

HIV treatment outcomes

COVID-19 may have an impact on HIV treatment cascade outcomes. Visits with healthcare professionals may be put on hold due to social distancing measures. Therefore, diagnosis of HIV may be delayed due to health care providers and patients putting HIV testing on hold. Linkage to HIV care may also be delayed due to COVID-19 patients being prioritized (Jiang et al., 2020). These delays will undoubtedly affect patients' engagement in care. Algarin et al. found that 10 out of 12 older adults living with HIV who had appointments had kept their appointments and the same proportion who knew they had a case manager had contacted their case manager. However, this estimate does not capture older adults who have not made appointments and are who are not aware of their case manager.

Patients' engagement in care may also impact antiretroviral therapy (ART) adherence. Higher adherence has been linked to greater viral suppression (Shiau et al., 2020) and lower ART adherence can cause adverse physical and mental health outcomes (Jiang et al., 2020). Viral suppression rates among older adults living with HIV may also be attenuated due to lower ART adherence and routine schedules being disrupted. Changes to viral suppression rates might not be seen immediately but may be a delayed effect that health care providers should be on the lookout for.

Author SBW is Chief of Infectious Diseases at an immunology clinic located in Columbia, South Carolina. Telehealth was quickly adapted in this clinic with respect to continuation of HIV care. This may improve access to care for some older adults, especially those with limited mobility. However, some older populations may struggle with the technology and prefer in-person visits. As telehealth is implemented, special attention needs to be paid to the specific needs of the older population.

Psychosocial challenges

Loneliness (Greene et al., 2018) and social isolation are key factors that affect older adults living with HIV. Depression is also a common mental health challenge among this population with approximately four in ten older adults having symptoms of major depression (Grov et al., 2010). Lonely older adults living with HIV have a higher likelihood of reporting depression and report fewer social connections (Greene et al., 2018). Stigma is also another factor that some older adults living with HIV face. They may undergo HIV-related stigma and ageism, which may limit access to social support from a variety of avenues including family and social structures (Cahill & Valadez, 2013). Now these factors may be exacerbated by the COVID-19 pandemic. There is a growing interest in how COVID-19 may impact the mental health of individuals (Joska et al., 2020). Indeed, COVID-19, it's potential impact on health, social isolation and the subsequent economic hardship has had a negative effect on stress (Algarin et al., 2020) and mental health. In addition, new barriers have been created for populations who have mental health and substance use challenges (Kaiser Family Foundation, 2020). Stigma has also been associated with COVID-19, which can increase the risk of exclusion, depression, and access to health care (Mayo Clinic, 2020).

Long-term HIV survivors

"Long-term HIV survivors" refer to people who have lived with HIV for several years. Some long-term HIV survivors have faced a myriad of challenges such as posttraumatic stress disorder (PTSD), housing and financial security, comorbidities and premature aging (Birnstengel, 2020). They have a higher likelihood of mortality and morbidity (Gebo, 2006). In addition, prolonged exposure to ART may lead to increased risk of adverse health outcomes, including heart disease (Deeks & Phillips, 2009). Nevertheless, the impact of COVID-19 can add significantly to the concerns of long-term survivors of

HIV through exacerbating mental health effects, financial uncertainty, and additional comorbidity.

Vulnerable populations

HIV and COVID-19 rates are higher among specific groups. For example, Black populations are disproportionately affected by HIV and mortality due to COVID-19. In South Carolina, where our clinic is located, Black populations comprise 27% of the state's total population but account for 68% of people living with HIV (South Carolina Department of Health and Environmental Control, 2020a) and 45% of reported COVID-19 cases (South Carolina Department of Health and Environmental Control, 2020b). Research has shown that LGBTQ populations are also at increased risk for complications due to COVID-19 (Human Rights Campaign, 2020). Specifically, they are less likely to have access to medical care and live in poverty. Therefore, LGBTQ populations of older adults will also be at an even higher risk of morbidity and mortality as a result of COVID-19. Recent research has called for studies on COVID-19 in HIV patients especially among older men who have sex with men (MSM) populations (Blanco et al., 2020).

Conclusions

Some older adults living with HIV face many challenges, which have been exacerbated by the COVID-19 pandemic. These include staying engaged with HIV care, mental health and physical health challenges. At present, long term outcome data do not exist to know how COVID impacts HIV prevention efforts, diagnosis, treatment outcomes and viral loads. Therefore, this is an area that needs to be studied and monitored continuously. The needs of long-term HIV survivors and additionally vulnerable groups (for example, Black populations, older MSM) should also be considered. In spite of the challenges faced, older adults living with HIV are a resilient group. Social workers and healthcare providers should not forget about this vulnerable population as older adults living with HIV navigate uncertainty with regards to HIV treatment and care, and their overall well-being in the midst of the COVID-19 pandemic.

Monique J. Brown

http://orcid.org/0000-0001-9552-244X

Sharon B. Weissman

Funding

This work was supported by the National Institute of Mental Health [K01MH115794].

References

Algarin, A. B., Varas-Rodríguez, E., Valdivia, C., Fennie, K. P., Larkey, L., Hu, N., & Ibañez, G. E. (2020). Symptoms, stress, and HIV-related care among older people living with HIV during the COVID-19 pandemic, Miami, Florida. *AIDS and Behavior*, 1–3. https://doi.org/10.1007/s10461-020-02869-3

Birnstengel, G. (2020). *Long-term survivors of HIV/AIDS reflect on what they've witnessed and endured.* https://www.pbs.org/newshour/health/long-term-survivors-of-hiv-aids-reflect-on-what-theyve-witnessed-and-endured

Blanco, J. L., Ambrosioni, J., Garcia, F., Martínez, E., Soriano, A., Mallolas, J., & Miro, J. M. (2020). COVID-19 in patients with HIV: Clinical case series. *The Lancet HIV*, *7*(5), e314–e316. https://doi.org/10.1016/s2352-3018(20)30111-9

Cahill, S., & Valadez, R. (2013). Growing older with HIV/AIDS: New public health challenges. *American Journal of Public Health*, *103*(3), e7–e15. https://doi.org/10.2105/AJPH.2012.301161

Deeks, S. G., & Phillips, A. N. (2009). HIV infection, antiretroviral treatment, ageing, and non-AIDS related morbidity. *BMJ*, *338*(jan26 2), a3172. https://doi.org/10.1136/bmj.a3172

Gebo, K. A. (2006). HIV and aging: Implications for patient management. *Drugs and Aging, 23* (11), 897–913. https://doi.org/10.2165/00002512-200623110-00005

Greene, M., Hessol, N. A., Perissinotto, C., Zepf, R., Hutton Parrott, A., Foreman, C., Whirry, R., Gandhi, M., & John, M. (2018). Loneliness in older adults living with HIV. *AIDS and Behavior*, *22*(5), 1475–1484. https://doi.org/10.1007/s10461-017-1985-1

Grov, C., Golub, S. A., Parsons, J. T., Brennan, M., & Karpiak, S. E. (2010). Loneliness and HIV-related stigma explain depression among older HIV-positive adults. *AIDS Care*, *22*(5), 630–639. https://doi.org/10.1080/09540120903280901

Human Rights Campaign. (2020). *The lives and livelihoods of many in the LGBTQ community are at risk amidst COVID-19 crisis.* https://www.hrc.org/resources/the-lives-and-livelihoods-of-many-in-the-lgbtq-community-are-at-risk-amidst

Jiang, H., Zhou, Y., & Tang, W. (2020). Maintaining HIV care during the COVID-19 pandemic. *The Lancet HIV*, *7*(5), e308–e309. https://doi.org/10.1016/s2352-3018(20)30105-3

Johns Hopkins University. (2020). *Coronavirus resource center.* https://coronavirus.jhu.edu/map.html

Joska, J. A., Andersen, L., Rabie, S., Marais, A., Ndwandwa, E. S., Wilson, P., & Sikkema, K. J. (2020). COVID-19: Increased risk to the mental health and safety of women living with HIV in South Africa. *AIDS and Behavior*, 1–3. https://doi.org/10.1007/s10461-020-02897-z

Kaiser Family Foundation. (2020). *The Implications of COVID-19 for mental health and substance use.* https://www.kff.org/health-reform/issue-brief/the-implications-of-covid-19-for-mental-health-and-substance-use/

Mayo Clinic. (2020). *COVID-19 (coronavirus) stigma: What it is and how to reduce it.* https://www.mayoclinic.org/diseases-conditions/coronavirus/in-depth/coronavirus-stigma/art-20484278

Shiau, S., Krause, K. D., Valera, P., Swaminathan, S., & Halkitis, P. N. (2020). The burden of COVID-19 in people living with HIV: A syndemic perspective. *AIDS and Behavior*, 1–6. https://doi.org/10.1007/s10461-020-02871-9

South Carolina Department of Health and Environmental Control. (2020a). *An epidemiologic profile of HIV and AIDS in South Carolina 2019.* https://scdhec.gov/sites/default/files/media/document/2019-Epi-Profile.pdf

South Carolina Department of Health and Environmental Control. (2020b). *SC demographic data (COVID-19).* https://www.scdhec.gov/infectious-diseases/viruses/coronavirus-disease-2019-covid-19/sc-demographic-data-covid–19

Serving LGBTQ+/SGL Elders during the Novel Corona Virus (COVID-19) Pandemic: Striving for Justice, Recognizing Resilience

Dear Editor,

The World Health Organization (WHO) declared the Novel Corona Virus (COVID-19) outbreak a global pandemic on March 11 of this year (WHO, 2020). In the time since, it has become clear that the virus carries the greatest risk for older individuals and those living with ongoing medical conditions (CDC, 2020). As a result of a lifetime of discrimination due to who they love and how they identify, lesbian, gay, bisexual, transgender, queer, and same-gender-loving (LGBTQ+/SGL) older adults are more likely to experience risk factors associated with serious illness and poor outcomes related to COVID-19. It is also not the first time they have encountered a pandemic that threatened their communities and comparisons between the AIDS crisis and COVID-19 have emerged in recent news (Bernstein, 2020). Against the backdrop of the pandemic, associated societal ageism and continued social distancing, Black Lives Matter protests broke out across the U.S. 2 months after WHO's declaration, sparked by police brutality targeting Black and African American communities in the wake of George Floyd's death. These two contemporaneous and ongoing social issues have illuminated existing disparities in life, health, and opportunity as well as the insidious and interlocking social causes of these injustices. In light of this unprecedented moment, we find ourselves taking stock and asking what it means to serve LGBTQ+/SGL elders in the context of COVID-19, across intersections of identity and interlocking dimensions of research, policy, and practice.

The COVID-19 pandemic has revealed existing health disparities among older adults while also exacerbating inequities in service access. The virus is known to carry the greatest risk of severe illness for older adults and those with underlying medical conditions and older adults of color have been disproportionately impacted (CDC, 2020). Of the 2.7 million LGBTQ+/SGL adults age 50 and older in the U.S., one-fifth of which are people of color, many are at higher medical risk, as mounting evidence indicates disparities in general health, disability, and chronic conditions associated with past experiences of discrimination and stigma among other factors (Fredriksen-Goldsen et al., 2019; MAP & SAGE, 2020). Prior to the pandemic, this population had also reported unique barriers to accessing care stemming from a lack of financial access, fears of discrimination or judgment, and concerns over one's safety and ability to find community, particularly in long-term care settings (Fredriksen-

Goldsen et al., 2019; Putney et al., 2018) and to the greatest degree among older adults of color and transgender individuals (MAP & SAGE, 2020). Limited access to health care due to interpersonal reasons as well as religious freedom policies allowing discriminatory practices, may mean that LGBTQ +/SGL elders are unlikely to access virus testing and medical care required during the pandemic. LGBTQ+/SGL older adults are also more likely to live alone and report social isolation, compared to heterosexual and cisgender counterparts (The Fenway Institute, 2020). Although often necessary, shelter-in-place and social distancing guidelines will likely deepen these issues along with the negative mental and physical health outcomes associated with isolation and loneliness. Additionally, almost a quarter of these older adults report that they have no one to call in case of an emergency (MAP & SAGE, 2020), meaning that they may have to choose between the safety of social distancing and attaining basic needs, such as groceries and medications during the pandemic. In light of these factors, a constellation of issues related to COVID-19 are anticipated as new or exacerbated concerns among this population. Existing disparities also vary in type and severity across social identities and positionings, and are particularly apparent among black (Woody, 2014) and other individuals of color and trans-identified folks. Thus, we have reached a stage at which subgroup analyses are needed in order to understand the perspectives, lives, needs, and strengths of LGBTQAI+/SGL older adults more fully as we gain a clearer picture of this population's relative experiences with COVID-19.

As social workers and service providers, we are guided by practice approaches that are person-centered, strength-based, and trauma-informed. Our values push us to strive for the equitable achievement of life, health, and opportunity. These skills and goals enable us to engage across levels of practice to take action. As a discipline, we must act in solidarity with those most impacted in times of crisis and with accountability to the goals of the profession. This requires that we build awareness of and celebrate sexual and gender diversity and anti-racist praxis. Advocacy must occur to counter policies allowing for healthcare discrimination against LGBTQ+/SGL individuals who already faced significant barriers to care. At an individual level, we can care and advocate for the LGBTQ+/SGL elders in our lives while limiting the risks of transmission that are within our scope of control. We can reach out to elders to combat social isolation, foster connection, and maintain a sense of community. Limiting direct contact and protecting ourselves from harm can be difficult for social workers; we strive to be the good person in the storm and many of us came to this profession out of a felt duty to serve. However, when possible, these steps are crucial in order to protect particularly those most vulnerable among us. From a trauma-informed perspective, not only are we living through a collective societal trauma, but we are also seeing the exacerbation of preexisting traumas, triggered by isolation, fear, and uncertainty. Many LGBTQ+/SGL older adults have survived high rates of violence, discrimination, and victimization over the course of their lives and many also carry painful memories of the AIDS crisis, another pandemic wrought with injustice and inequality. Professional empathy and person-centered understandings of marginalized clients' lives and experiences are needed now more than ever.

We have called attention to disparities and need among this population, a message only deepened by the current context, but a balance of strengths-based and resilience-centering narratives is also required in order to inspire hope and create change. May we be guided by the resilience and perseverance of LGBTQ+/SGL older adults themselves. Despite existing risk factors and historical trauma, our elders show strength through spiritual resilience, activism, solidarity across a wide range of identities, high rates of caregiving, and an uncanny ability to create and maintain chosen families and communities (Fredriksen-Goldsen et al., 2019; Woody, 2014). Let us act as an empowering influence by supporting and building upon such strengths as we simultaneously seek to right the wrongs of history.

Sarah Jen

Dan Stewart

Imani Woody

References

Bernstein, J. (2020, April). For H.I.V. survivors, a feeling of weary déjà vu. *New York Times.* https://www.nytimes.com/2020/04/08/style/coronavirus-hiv.html

Centers for Disease Control and Prevention. (2020, June). *People who are at increased risk for severe illness.* https://www.cdc.gov/coronavirus/2019-ncov/need-extra-precautions/people-at-increased-risk.html

Fredriksen-Goldsen, K. I., Jen, S., & Muraco, A. (2019). Iridescent life course: LGBTQ aging research and blueprint for the future-A systematic review. *Gerontology, 65*(3), 253–274. https://doi.org/10.1159/000493559

Movement Advancement Project & Advocacy and Services for LGBT Elders (MAP, SAGE). (2020). *LGBT older people & COVID-19: Addressing higher risk, social isolation, and discrimination.* https://www.lgbtmap.org/file/2020%20LGBTQ%20Older%20Adults%20COVID.pdf

Putney, J. M., Keary, S., Hebert, N., Krinsky, L., & Halmo, R. (2018). ""Fear Runs Deep:" The Anticipated Needs of LGBT Older Adults in Long-Term Care" The anticipated needs of LGBT older adults in long-term care. Journal of gerontological social work, 61(8),887-907. doi:10.1080/01634372.2018.1508109

The Fenway Institute. (2020). *Coronavirus, COVID-19, and considerations for people living with HIV and LGBTQIA+ people.* https://www.lgbtagingcenter.org/resources/pdfs/C19MC-9_COVID-19and-LGBTQIA-and-People-Living-with-HIV-Brief_final2_links.pdf

The World Health Organization. (2020). *Timeline of WHO's response to COVID-19.* https://www.who.int/news-room/detail/29-06-2020-covidtimeline

Woody, I. (2014). Aging Out: A Qualitative Exploration of Ageism and Heterosexism Among Aging African American Lesbians and Gay Men. Journal of Homosexuality, 61(1),145-165. doi:10.1080/00918369.2013.835603

Older Adults and Covid 19: Social Justice, Disparities, and Social Work Practice

Carole Cox

ABSTRACT

The Covid- 19 pandemic has brought immense challenges to almost every country as it spreads throughout their populations. Foremost among these challenges is the heightened awareness of inequalities in society and the immense toll that the virus has on the most vulnerable. Globally, older people are the most at risk of getting the virus and dying from the it. Yet, although age is a significant contributor, it is its interaction with other factors, chronic conditions, poverty, and race that makes it a strong determinant. These factors reflect disparities and systemic social injustices that interact to increase the vulnerability of older adults. This paper discusses the many roles that social work, with its focus on social change, injustice, and vulnerable groups can intervene at many levels of practice and with specific groups to alleviate these fundamental disparities.

The Covid- 19 pandemic has brought immense challenges to almost every country as it spreads throughout their populations. Foremost among these challenges is the heightened awareness of inequalities in society and the immense toll that the virus has on the most vulnerable. Globally, older people are the most at risk of getting the virus and dying from the it. Yet, although age is a significant contributor, it is its interaction with other factors, chronic conditions, poverty, and race that makes it a strong determinant. Each of these factors, as they intersect with health care, housing, employment, and education intersect to make specific groups of older adults at increased risk. Together, they underscore the relationship of inequality and vulnerability to the right to life itself. As summed up by the Secretary General of the United Nations (Guiterras, 2020) "The right to life and duty to protect life; the right to health and access to care; and freedom of movement are "frontline in the current pandemic."

These rights and duties are embedded in the goals of the social work profession whose mission is to promote social justice and social change with and on behalf of clients, particularly the vulnerable and oppressed in society (NASW Code of Ethics, 2017). Focusing on the situation in the United States, this paper focuses on key social justice disparities that increase the vulnerability of older adults to Covid-19 and the ways in which social work interventions can work to alleviate these fundamental disparities.

Social determinants of Covid-19

Age

Although criteria for vulnerability may differ among countries, one common characteristic is its disproportionate impact on older people. More than 95% of the people dying from the virus in Europe were 65 years and older (Human Rights Watch, 2020) while, similarly in the United States, as of March, 2020, more than 8% of the deaths were those 65 and older with the mortality rate highest for those for those over 85, (CDC, 2020).

Accompanying these rates has been an increase in ageism, discrimination against older persons. Ageism has been surging globally as older persons are the group most likely to be hospitalized and to die as a result of Covid-19. Age alone is not a factor, the living situations of older people in congregate facilities as well as underlying medical conditions that impact their immunity, increase the risk of Covid-19. Unfortunately, as with other "isms" ageism has many ramifications affecting older adults during the pandemic.

Ageism perpetuates negative stereotypes that describe older people as frail with diminished status creating burdens on society, have been spread by media in many countries (Ayalon et al., 2020). Such attitudes and beliefs undervalue the contributions of older adults and may even impact access to services and supports, particularly when resources are scarce. Ageism also suggests that it is mainly older adults who struggle most with isolation, ignoring how isolation and loneliness affects all age groups (Gerontological Society of America, 2020).

Ageism is present in the development of vaccines against the virus. Although older people are disproportionately affected by the virus, they are not necessarily included in clinical trials. Guidance offered by the F.D.A. on participation is not binding and trials frequently set age limits, often excluding those over 65. Safety issues, as well as expediency for the researcher, the beliefs that older people lack technology, and are not fluent with computers, are commonly given as reasons for exclusion (NY Times, June 21, 2020). Without being included, the effectiveness of vaccines or treatments for older adults cannot be known.

Race and ethnicity

African Americans, Latinos and other minority groups are disproportionately affected by the virus with higher rates of hospitalization or death from the virus (Kaiser Family Foundation, 2020). The risks for the illness among these groups is compounded by poverty, poor and crowded housing, lower paying and more stressful employment. The increased incidence of underlying chronic health conditions, cardiac disease, chronic metabolic disease, hypertension, and obesity are major risk factors for racial and ethnic minority elderly (CDC, 2020). Discrimination in the health care sector itself also increases the risk as racial and ethnic minority persons report more negative experiences with providers and are less likely than whites to receive quality care (Artiga et al., 2020). Consequently, they are less likely than other groups to delay going for treatment or to avoid it completely. Thus, when they do go for care, they are more likely to be in advanced stages of the virus, to be hospitalized, and to die from it.

Social workers must work toward assuring more equitable health care that protects older adults. Advocating for increased insurance coverage, including the expansion of the Affordable Care Act and Medicaid, can be of particular benefit to low income older adults. Assuring that all persons have correct information with materials in languages that they can read is a prerogative to utilization. Working with other public health personnel, social workers can aid in dispersing education about the virus to local community groups and programs.

The disparities associated with race are clearly represented in the impact of Covid-19 on nursing homes. Across the country, homes with larger proportions of black and Latino residents have been twice as likely to have the virus as homes that have a majority of white residents (NY Times, May 21, 2020). Nursing homes, similar to schools, tend to be segregated according to the neighborhoods they are in. Those in predominantly black and Latino areas serve primarily these residents. As these homes are often in urban areas, are very large, and tend to score worse by nursing home regulators, they are more likely to have residents who contract the virus and die from it. These homes are also less likely to have protective gear for staff and to have staff who work in multiple facilities, further increasing the likelihood of spreading the virus.

The disparities among nursing homes reflect the racial injustice in our society. Advocating for major policy changes that increase the quality of these homes and thus the standard of care that they offer is essential. Immediate concerns such as increasing staff and providing them with necessary protective equipment is a beginning step for further reforms. Partnering with other groups such as nursing home ombudsmen and family associations, social workers can help to develop strong advocacy coalitions that lead to long lasting reforms and improvements in care.

Poverty

Poverty increases the risk of Covid-19 as it is associated with poorer health status and living conditions. The risk is magnified for older adults whose age alone increases their vulnerability. Data from the Kaiser Family Foundation (2018) show 14% of persons age 65 and above below 100% of the poverty line ($11,756 per year) and 42% below 200% of the poverty line ($23, 512 per year). When separating poverty by race and ethnicity, the proportion living below 200% of poverty is significantly higher for black (60.3%) and Hispanic older adults (65.5%) than it is for white (37.2%).

The intersectionality of race, income, and health threatens the well-being and lives of these persons. With the pandemic, many community and senior centers have closed, removing the common places where they may have had nutritious meals. Without being able to follow a physician's dietary advice, there is an increased risk of aggravating conditions such as diabetes and hypertension (Brookings Institute, 2020). Low income, with increasing financial demands, motivates many to continue to work, even in high risk jobs where they are vulnerable to contacting the virus and spreading it.

At the micro level, social workers can assure that persons apply for all potential benefits. As well as financial support, this must provide links with local food banks and meal delivery programs. At the mezzo level, social workers may assist programs in identifying those at risk and developing services to help them. The macro level demands advocating for significant policy changes that recognize and erase the inequities that are contributing to poverty and its resulting vulnerabilities.

Social isolation

The requirement that social isolation is key to confronting the virus has an immense impact on older adults. Without contact, these persons are placed at increased risk of emotional and psychological problems. Being isolated from social networks that include friends and family can result in depression and distress that impact both mental and physical health and lead to an increased risk of mortality (Holt-Lunstad et al., 2015; Taylor et al., 2018). In addition, the risk of developing dementia has also been linked to a lack of socialization and engagement (Sundström et al., 2020). Particularly important is the finding that feelings of loneliness in itself may act as a risk factor for dementia (Holwerda et al., 2014).

Social isolation can indirectly also contribute to poorer health status. Changes in food and nutrition associated with decreased access and availability can impact cardiac conditions while sheltering in place can result in less exercise contributing to weakness, frailty, and falls (Steinman et al., 2020). Without others to interact with, symptoms, both behavioral and physical, including those associated with Covid-19, may go unnoticed.

Interventions to combat isolation and loneliness are critical for both physical and mental health. On the micro level, social workers' counseling with isolated persons can play an important supportive role. Telephone and video calls are an immediate way of connecting, assessing functioning, and maintaining relationships. Traditional support groups can be adapted into virtual groups so that participants can continue to share and engage with each other. As an example, the Circle of Friends program in St. Louis moved from a traditional group to a telehealth delivery program that can also continue to be used after the pandemic (Berg-Weger & Morley, 2020).

At the mezzo level, social workers can help to assure that agencies have such programs and that volunteers or recruited and trained to offer appropriate counseling with older adults. As an example, Dorot in New York City, has a telephone bank composed of students who talk once or twice a week with seniors living alone. The program replaces traditional original home visits and provides important connections with the older clients (Dorot, 2020).

The challenge at the macro level is to advocate for policies that reduce the impact of social isolation and loneliness on older adults. Joining with other stakeholders, social workers can advocate for improving access to services that reduce isolation and foster connectedness. As an, example The Coalition to End Social Isolation and Loneliness works for legislation to improve health and services for isolated vulnerable populations and obtain additional funds for services for older adults. Participating in this type of coalition can bring further attention to the factors contributing to loneliness and ways of alleviating it.

Home care

Nearly six million Americans rely on home care services, more than live in nursing homes and assisted living combined (Landers, 2016). In 2016, there were 12,200 home health agencies in the US serving more than 3 million people through the Medicare home health benefit (MEDPAC, 2019). The average cost for homecare, 22.50 USD an hour, is much less than nursing home care. (Genworth, 2020).

However, home care workers struggle, making an average of 11.52 USD an hour (PHI, 2019). They typically have no health insurance and half rely on public assistance, even though during the Covid-19 pandemic, they were declared essential workers. However, even as essential, they may actually be spreading the virus. Nearly 60% belong to racial or ethnic minority groups, with a median age of 49. Many work at several homes without protective clothing, have little professional training, experience stress, and do not receive regular testing. All of these factors compromise the care they offer as well as increase their risk of transmitting the virus.

The original Medicare benefit did not include prevention or care for those who were chronically ill and thus was restricted in its assistance to persons with Covid-19. In March, 2020, Congress passed the Coronavirus Aid, Relief, and Economic Security Act (CARES). Under the ACT, Medicare' home health benefit is expanded as it permits nurse practitioners and physician assistants, rather than demanding a physician's referral to order services. Isolation, rather than strict homebound criteria, are also considered as eligibility criteria for care. The Act allows telehealth so that persons can communicate with doctors without traveling out of their homes although agencies are not reimbursed for the service. This expansion of home care should relieve the demand for institutional care while concomitantly, supporting the right of older adults to remain in their own homes in the community.

Given the critical role of home health workers in community care, their status and skills must be strengthened. Developing skills along with higher salaries can alleviate the pressure to attend to many clients, reducing their stress as well as the risk that they may be transmitting the virus. Likewise, quality home care is an essential part of long term support services while competent trained workers may help to reduce the need for nursing home placement. Social workers in health care settings are in key positions to advocate for policies that strengthen the roles of home care workers and consequently improve the care they offer to older adults.

Technological support

Technology can act as a vital support for older adults. It can be used for counseling, telehealth, and for virtual support groups. Data from the United States indicate that two-thirds of adults 65 and older use the internet (Nash, 2019). However, only about half of persons 65 and older have broadband at home (Pew Research Center, 2017). Disparities by income show 62% of those with incomes of 75,000 USD or more have a computer in their home in comparison to only 16% of those with incomes less than 30,000 USD a year (Pew Research Center, 2017).

Efforts to increase the availability of digital technology to older adults are important as the internet can help to alleviate isolation as well as be used for telehealth and even activities such as online shopping. As well as assisting older adults, technology can also relieve caregiver stress, as the internet can be used to monitor their relatives when they are alone.

Social work advocacy is an important tool for broadening the availability and accessibility of technology to older people living in the community. Advocacy efforts in New York City led to its partnering with T Mobile to disperse 10,000 tablets and internet connections to over 10,000 seniors living in New York City Public Housing. The program also provides free technology training to the recipients with the ultimate goal of helping them to stay connected. (NYC CTO, 2020).

Nursing home care

In the United States, nearly 26,000 nursing home residents have died from Covid-19 and more than 60,000 have been ill with it (CDC, 2020). Reasons for the outbreak include poor testing regimes, poor protective equipment, little regulation of staff, and failure to separate infected residents from others. Such high death rates suggest that governments are lax to respond to health threats impacting older adults and their rights to security and appropriate health care and services (Human Rights Watch, 2020).

As a means of controlling the virus, one of the initial policies in facilities has been to restrict visitors. In March,2020, the Center for Medicare and Medicaid Services (CMS) issued guidance that facilities should restrict the visitation of all visitors except for certain compassionate care situations, such as an end-of-life situation. Although the policies exempted visits for those near the end of life, many facilities restricted even these visits. Consequently, persons have been left to die alone while families' requests to visit are denied.

The compromised health of residents and the settings of facilities contributes to the spread and severity of the virus. However, in the urgency to restrain the virus, national policy ignored basic prevention measures such as trained staff, proper equipment, reporting the number of residents with Covid-19, and the testing of all residents and staff. The lack of transparency in nursing home that keeps family members from learning of the status of their relative or of the impact of the disease on the home is a major stressor to families (AARP, 2020).

At the micro level, social workers can provide counseling to residents and to their relatives to support them in coping with the virus. At the meso level, social workers, cognizant of the needs of the home, the resident, and the families can advocate for more testing, staff, and more means for them to communicate with the resident, with greater transparency about resident status.

At the macro level, policies that support the rights of residents and families are essential. The factors leading to the vulnerability of residents must be identified and dealt with so that homes do not increase the vulnerability of residents. Advocating for reforms that include adequate staffing for a health care crisis, space for social distancing and separation of those that require isolation, and transparency regarding a nursing home's quality are important issues in which social workers can use join with others to advocate for change.

Special needs groups

Persons with dementia

Persons with dementia and their caregivers face particular challenges with regards to Covid-19. Due to their illness, they may ignore recommendations regarding face coverings and social distancing, isolating, have difficulty monitoring symptoms and are at risk of being doubly stigmatized (Brown et al., 2020). This stigmatization can jeopardize their receipt of scarce resources such as ventilators and intensive care beds. and being overlooked by health professionals and health systems that are not trained in caring for them (Milken Institute, 2020).

Persons who have been living in the community often depend on an array of services such as home delivered meals and home attendants. If these services are unavailable and they lack informal supports, there is an increased risk institutionalization. Technological supports that can aid other older adults may not be accessible to those with dementia, further compromising their ability to live at home. If they are forced to be hospitalized or move to an institutional, they can easily be overwhelmed by the transition.

Social workers have critical roles in supporting persons with dementia in the community and linking them with services that may enable them to remain at home. Through counseling and information, many be able to follow guidelines and simple instructions. Micro interventions must include working with the families so that they are knowledgeable about the potential impact that the virus may have on their relative. This should involve helping them to develop plans if visits and services are disrupted and they are unable to provide needed care.

At the meso level, social workers are important in helping agencies develop services for this special population, assuring that staff are trained in working with persons with dementia. Working with institutions, social workers can intervene to facilitate the transitions process from the community, reducing the disruption and stress it can cause. Macro work must focus on policies that strengthen support services for persons with dementia and their families. This includes more options for community care so that many can remain at home and families receive supports that enable them as caregivers. Attention must also be given to the development of residential facilities that are specific to the care of persons with dementia so that their specific needs can be better addressed.

Caregivers

There are approximately 34 million people acting as caregivers for an older adult in the United States (Family Caregiver Alliance, 2019). The demands associated with the role have intensified with COVID-19. As described by Lightfoot and Moore (2020) caregivers are subject to social isolation, potential burnout without access to usual supports, limited access to technology, social distancing demanded by health care facilities, and financial hardship.

As well as offering counseling and support to these caregivers, social workers must become active in advocating for long term support services (LTSS) that can benefit their relative and reduced their own strain. Medicaid is the largest payer of LTSS in the United States covering 42% of all LTSS services (Congressional Research Service, 2018). However, not all state programs recognize caregivers and their needs for assistance. The advocacy skills and involvement of social workers, joining with other stakeholders, such as the National Alliance on Caregiving, can work toward major policy changes that recognize and strengthen the roles of family caregivers.

Grandparent caregivers

There are approximately 2.7 million grandparents in the United States who are responsible for the primary care of their grandchildren without any other adult present (U.S. Census, 2018).For every 1 child in foster care, there are 20 being raised by grandparents (Wiltz, 2018). The primary reasons for assuming care for the children are death, substance abuse, mental health issues, disabilities, incarceration, and military deployment, with almost half of the children in these households in poverty.

Kinship care has many benefits for children as it maintains familial bonds and provides children with a sense of security. It helps minimize trauma and loss associated with separation from parents. In comparison to those in non-kin foster care, children in kinship care change schools less frequently, have fewer behavioral problems, and if reunited with their birth parents, are less likely to enter foster care again (Bavier, 2011). The majority of these grandparents have no legal relationship to the children and are informal caregivers who thus may not be eligible for all benefits (Annie & Casey Foundation, 2017).

Health is a concern in the lives of custodial grandparents as chronic problems can affect their parenting ability. Preexisting conditions such as diabetes, hypertension, and heart disease can be exacerbated by the stress incumbent in the parenting role (Boetto, 2010). The transition into the parenting role can result in increased depression, obesity, and poorer-self rated health (Hughes et al, 2007). However, grandparents are often reluctant to seek care as any sign of frailty could make them vulnerable to losing their grandchildren (Cox, 2009).

The Covid-19 pandemic has added an extra strain on these caregivers. Given the propensity of underlying conditions, they are vulnerable to the virus while worries about caring for their grandchildren may lead to the denial of symptoms and treatment. Isolation presents a further strain as it can impede their ability to get food and other supplies. Without assistance, shopping can be difficult, particularly if it entails always being accompanied by children, even to food pantries.

School age children suddenly dealing with online learning pose new challenges to grandparents. Many grandparents lack skills in the technology necessary for online learning increasing their stress as they try to help children with schoolwork. Adolescents, eager to socialize with friends, can cause further strains as grandparents attempt to balance their grandchildren's' needs for independence with the threat of their bringing the virus home.

Social work interventions are important for supporting this population. At the micro level, social workers provide education and counseling that assist grandparents in coping with the stresses associated with the virus. At the mezzo level, they can link grandparents with support groups that do not necessarily demand video access. Empowering grandparents to feel comfortable in discussing their concerns with teachers can strengthen their relationships with schools (Todd, 2020). For many, this offers a new opportunity to be positively engaged in their children's lives.

The CARES Act (April,2020) designated some funding specifically for grandparent headed families. However, the allocation of these funds depends to a large extent on local advocacy and the ability of advocates to raise awareness of the need for supports for these families (Generations United, 2020). Joining with other community groups such as state and local kinship care organizations that lobby for funds and programs, social work advocates can use their skills to underscore the roles that these grandparents play and the resources that can assist them.

Conclusions

Rosa Kornfeld-Matte, the independent expert on the human rights of older persons has stressed the particular concerns of older adults during the Covid-19 pandemic and the issues caused by poverty, limited access to services, and the conditions in care homes and the urgent need to ensure support services with heightening the risk to care providers (OHCHR, 2020).

Covid-19 underscores the many inequalities impacting the lives and well-being of older adults. Race, ethnicity, and poverty all intersect to increase the chances of both getting and dying from the virus. Together these factors contribute to age discrimination which in itself can easily marginalize older adults and further accentuate disparities that threaten their rights and lives.

The predisposing conditions that cause older people to be most susceptible to the virus reflect the disparities in our society. Heart disease, hypertension, and diabetes are overrepresented in the older minority populations while their access to health care is often limited. These injustices that contribute to their susceptibility to Covid-19 also increase their chances of dying from it. The nursing homes caring for these older adults are likely to be the ones with the fewer resources and trained staff. Consequently, the same factors that predispose to the virus also predispose to mortality.

Social work interventions to reduce the systemic disparities impacting older adults in the midst of the Covid-19 pandemic are essential. As well as working to alleviate the predisposing conditions that threaten older adults, efforts must also be made to improve the quality of those caring for them. Increasing the training and supports and the wages for home attendants and nurses aides are important steps in developing a better trained and safer workforce. Advocating for more caregiver supports, including technology in the home, can lead to changes that ease caregiver stress, reduce isolation and enable more persons to remain in the community. In addition, social workers can use their advocacy skills to press for policies that improve and ease the transition process when persons with dementia must move from the community to an institution.

Social isolation can be particularly threatening for older adults and efforts must be made to minimize it. Daily telephone calls, virtual visits and support groups, even by telephone, can help to reduce loneliness. In the same way, families need to be able to stay involved in the lives of nursing home residents so that connections are maintained. Social workers within the homes must work toward enabling these contacts whether though video calls or even limited visitation.

The effects of social isolation on grandparent headed families who face unique stresses associated with the virus can further jeopardize their well-being. The challenges of raising children without any supports and of dealing with schools are additional stresses for many families. Social work counseling is an important support, but grandparents must also be connected to services, including schools, and community programs and other resources such as online groups that can replace traditional support groups.

Social work education must underscore the ways in which lifetimes of disparity impact the individual and the aging process itself. Living with advantages and disadvantages cumulatively affects the later years, making those who are marginalized disproportionately vulnerable to morbidity and even death. As the pandemic has highlighted the interconnectedness of all individuals in society, education must address interventions and strategies that support people of all ages and groups with close attention given to the impact of policies and services on well-being.

Social work research on strategies that can dismantle barriers which continue to disenfranchise people is essential. Such research can help elucidate the factors that impede persons from seeking care as well as identify the challenges that they face. Incorporating the results of these studies into interventions can provide for more accessible and acceptable services and supports for all.

Covid-19 has underscored the ways that age discrimination, race and poverty interact to compound the impact of lifetimes of social injustices on older adults. The crisis associated with the pandemic presents incredible challenges as well as the opportunity for needed systemic changes that reduce social disparities. The result of such changes should last long after the pandemic as they serve to integrate all older adults into a just society. As a profession whose mission is grounded in social change, social work, with interventions that range from case to cause, has the ability to use its skills and processes to create a more equal society where policies, resources, and services benefit all groups, increasing the universal possibility of aging well.

References

AARP. (2020) *AARP is fighting the coronavirus crisis in nursing homes by demanding more transparency.* Washington, AARP. https://www.aarp.org/politics-society/advocacy/info-2020/jenkins-letter-coronavirus-nursing-home-reform-04-24.html

Annie, E., Casey Foundation. (2017). *Kids count data center, children in kinship care.* Author.

Artiga, S., Orgera, K., & Pham, O. (2020). *Disparities in health and health care: Key questions and answers.* Kaiser Family Foundation. https://www.kff.org/disparities-policy/issue-brief/disparities-in-health-and-health-care-five-key-questions-and-answers/

Ayalon, L., Chasteen, A., Diehl, M., Levy, B., Neupert, S., Rothermund, K., Tesch-Romer, C., & Wahl, H. (2020). Aging in times of the COVID-19 pandemic: Avoiding ageism and fostering intergenerational solidarity. *The Journals of Gerontology: Series B*, gbaa051. https://doi.org/10.1093/geronb/gbaa051

Bavier, R. (2011). Children residing with no parent present. *Children and Youth Services Review, 33*(10), 1891–1901. https://doi.org/10.1016/j.childyouth.2011.05.017

Berg-Weger, M., & Morley, J. (2020, April 14). Loneliness and social isolation in older adults during the Covid-19 pandemic: Implications for gerontological social work. *Journal of Nutrition, Health, and Aging, 24*(3), 1–3. https://doi.org/10.1007/s12603-020-1366-8

Boetto, H. (2010). Kinship care. *Family Matters, 85*, 60–67.

Brookings Institute. (2020) *For millions of low-income seniors, coronavirus is a food-security issue.* Washington, DC: Brookings. https://www.brookings.edu/blog/the-avenue/2020/03/16/for-millions-of-low-income-seniors-coronavirus-is-a-food-security-issue/

Brown, E., Kumar, S., Rajii, T., & Pollock, B. (2020). Anticipating and mitigating the impact of Covid 19 pandemic on Alzheimer's disease and related dementias. *The American Journal of Geriatric Psychiatry, 28*(7), 712–721. https://doi.org/10.1016/j.jagp.2020.04.010

CDC. (2020). *Covid view: A weekly summary.* Washington: Centers for Disease Control. Retrieved June 12, 2020, from https://www.cdc.gov/coronavirus/2019-ncov/covid-data/covidview/index.html

Congressional Research Service. (2018). Who pays for long-term services and supports? A fact sheet. Congressional Research Service. August. https://fas.org/sgp/crs/misc/IF10343.pdf.

Cox, C. (2009). Supporting grandparent-headed families. *The Prevention Researcher, 15*(3), 13–17.

Dorot. 2020, *Caring calls offers conversation and connection.* https://www.dorotusa.org/caring-calls-offers-conversation-and-connection

Family Caregiver Alliance (2019). *Caregiver statistics.* Family Caregiver Alliance. Retrieved June 2, 2020, from https://www.caregiver.org/print/23216

Genworth. (2020). *Cost of care, trends and insights.* Genworth. https://www.enworth.com/aging-and-you/finances/cost-of-care/cost-of-care-trends-and-insights.html

Gerontological Society of America. (2020). *Understanding Ageism and COVID-19.* Gerontological Society of America. https://www.geron.org/images/gsa/reframing/AgeismInfographic_final.pdf

Guiterras, A., (2020). *We are all in this together: Human rights and COVID-19- Response and recovery*. United Nations. https://www.un.org/en/un-coronavirus-communications-team /we-are-all-together-human-rights-and-covid-19-response-and

Holt-Lunstad, J., Smith, T. B., Baker, M., Harris, T., & Stephenson, D. (2015). Loneliness and social isolation as risk factors for mortality: A meta-analytic review. *Perspectives on Psychological Science, 10*(2), 227–237. https://doi.org/10.1177/1745691614568352

Holwerda, T. J., Deeg, D. J. H., Beekman, A. T. F., van Tilburg, T. G., Stek, M. L., Jonker, C., & Schoevers, R. A. (2014). Feelings of loneliness, but not social isolation, predict dementia onset: Results from the Amsterdam Study of the Elderly (AMSTEL). *Journal of Neurology, Neurosurgery, and Psychiatry, 85*(2), 135–142. https://doi.org/10.1136/jnnp-2012-302755

Hughes, M., Waite, L., & LaPierre, L. Y. (2007). The impact of caring for grandchildren on grandparents' health. *Journals of Gerontology Series B, 62*(2), 108–119. doi:https://doi.org/ 10.1093/geronb/62.2.S108

Human Rights Watch, April, 2020. *Rights risks to older people in Covid-19 response*. Human Rights Watch. https://www.hrw.org/news/2020/04/07/rights-risks-older-people-covid-19-response#

Kaiser Family Foundation. (2018). *How many seniors Live in Poverty?* Kaiser Family Foundation. https://www.kff.org/report-section/how-many-seniors-live-in-poverty-issue-brief

Kaiser Family Foundation. (2020). *Covid-19 cases by race/ethnicity*. Kaiser Family Foundation. www.kff.org/other/state-indicator/covid-19-cases-by-race-ethnicity/?currentTimeframe= 0&sortModel=%7BcolIdLocation sort asc%7D

Landers, S. (2016). The future of home health care, A strategic framework for optimizing value. *Home Health Care Management & Practice, 4*(3), 262–278. https://doi.org/10.1177/ 1084822316666368

Lightfoot, E., & Moore, T. (2020). Caregiving in times of uncertainty: Helping adult children of aging parents find support during the COVID-19 Outbreak. *Journal of Gerontological Social Work*, 1–11. https://doi.org/10.1080/01634372.2020.1769793

MEDPAC. (2019) *Medicare and the health care delivery system: Report to congress*. Medicare Payment Advisory Commission. http://www.medpac.gov/docs/default-source/reports/ jun19_medpac_reporttocongress_sec.pdf?sfvrsn=0

Milken Institute. (2020) *Recommendations to build a dementia-capable workforce and system amid COVID-19*. Milken Institute. https://milkeninstitute.org/sites/default/files/2020-05/ Recommendations%20to%20Build%20a%20Dementia-Capable%20Workforce%20and% 20System%20amid%20COVID-19_2020_05_04-FINAL%20.pdf

Nash, S. (2019) *Older adults and technology: Moving beyond the stereotypes*. Stanford Center on Longevity. http://longevity.stanford.edu/2019/05/30/older-adults-and-technology-moving-beyond-the-stereotypes/

National Association of Social Work. (2017) *NASW code of ethics*. National Association of Social Work. Retrieved June 4, 2020, from https://www.socialworkers.org/About/Ethics/ Code-of-Ethics/Code-of-Ethics-English

New York Times. (June 16, 2020a) Texas tries to balance local control with the threat of a pandemic. https://www.nytimes.com/2020/03/24/us/coronavirus-texas-patrick-abbott. html?0p19G=0

New York Times. (May 21, 2020b). *The striking racial divide in how Covid-19 has hit nursing homes*. https://www.nytimes.com/article/coronavirus-nursing-homes-racial-disparity.html? referringSource=articleShare

New York Times. (June 21, 2020c) Older adults may be left out of some Covid-19 trials. https:// www.nytimes.com/2020/06/19/health/vaccine-trials-elderly.html

NYC CTO (June 11, 2020) *City of New York Delivers 10,000 internet devices to older NYCHA residents*. Older Adults Technology Services. https://oats.org/nyc-mocto-city-of-new-york-delivers-10000-internet-devices-to-older-nycha-residents/

OHCHR. (2020). *Unacceptable – UN expert urges better protection of older persons facing the highest risk of the COVID-19 pandemic*. Office of High Commissioner on Human Rights. https://www.ohchr.org/EN/NewsEvents/Pages/DisplayNews.aspx?NewsID=25748&LangID=E

Pew Research Center. (2017). *Technology use among seniors*. Pew Research Center. https://www.pewresearch.org/internet/2017/05/17/technology-use-among-seniors/

PHI. (2019). *Workforce data center*. Direct Care Workers. Paraprofessional Healthcare Insitute. https://phinational.org/policy-research/workforce-data-center/

Steinman, M., Perry, L., & Perissinoot, C. (2020). Meeting the cae needs of older adults isolated at home during the Covid-19 pandemic. *Journal of American Medical Association, 180*(6), 819–820. https://doi.org/10.1001/jamainternmed.2020.1661

Sundström, A., Adolfsson, A., Nordin, M., & Adolfsson, R. (2020). Loneliness Increases the risk of all-cause dementia and Alzheimer's disease. *The Journals of Gerontology: Series B, 75*(5), 919-926. https://doi.org/10.1093/geronb/gbz139

Taylor, H., Taylor, R., Nguyen, A., & Chatters, L. (2018). Social isolation, depression and psychological distress among older adults. *Journal of Aging and Health, 30*(2), 229–246. https://doi.org/10.1177/0898264316673511

Todd, R. (2020). *Empowering families for distance learning in early childhood*. Edutopia. https://www.edutopia.org/article/empowering-families-distance-learning-early-childhood

U.S. Census. (2018). Older people living with grandchildren: 2012–2916. https://doi.org/10.1001/jamainternmed.2020.1661.

Wiltz, T. (2018). *Will the new foster care law give grandparents a hand?* PEW Trusts. https://www.pewtrusts.org/en/research-and-analysis/blogs/stateline/2018/06/05/will-the-new-foster-care-law-give-grandparents-a-hand

Part IV

COVID-19 and Health and Social Care

Self-Direction of Home and Community-Based Services in the Time of COVID-19

Kevin J. Mahoney

ABSTRACT

During the COVID-19 pandemic, nursing homes and assisted living facilities have accounted for over 20% of all infections, adult day care and other congregate sites have closed, and traditional home care agencies are facing staff shortages. In this environment, self-direction of home and community-based services, where the participant can hire their own staff and manage a budget that can be used for a broad range of goods and services including home modifications and assistive devices, is seen as a promising intervention. Using self-direction participants can minimize the number of people who enter their homes and pay close family and friends who were already providing many hours of informal care, and now may be unemployed. The Center for Medicare and Medicaid Services is encouraging this approach. This commentary presents information on how states have responded using the new CMS Toolkit by expanding who can be a paid caregiver, increasing budgets and broadening the kinds of items that can be purchased with budgets to include items like personal protective equipment and supports for telehealth. This Commentary concludes with policy and research questions regarding how the delivery of long-term services and supports (LTSS) may change as the world returns to "normal".

Over a fifth of the deaths from COVID-19 in the United States are tied to nursing homes or other long-term care facilities. Families are now reluctant to let their older members go to nursing facilities (Dolan & Hamilton, 2020).

As the pandemic continues, adult day centers are closing and home health agencies, already plagued by staff shortages, are finding that many workers are staying home to care for their own families or to protect themselves.

Concurrently, millions of Americans are laid off from their jobs and authorities have directed communities to "shelter in place".

In this environment, numerous states, with encouragement from the Centers for Medicare and Medicaid Services (CMS), are turning to self-direction of home and community-based services (HCBS). Under self-direction, available under Medicaid and via Veteran-Directed Care, participants can recruit and manage workers of their own choosing. Some programs allow participants to manage and control a budget which they can use, not only to employ care workers, but to pay for other supports. In self-direction, participants have support from a counselor to find creative ways to meet their needs, develop back-up plans, and locate necessary resources. Participants also have the help of financial management services agencies to pay bills, and act as payroll agents ensuring compliance with tax and labor requirements and preventing fraud.

Results from a randomized control experiment with thousands of participants have shown that self-direction reduces unmet needs, increases satisfaction with distinct aspects of care, improves health outcomes, and increases life satisfaction while leading to less financial, physical and emotional stress for families (Carlson et al., 2007). Availability of self-direction has grown steadily. By 2015 every state had at least one Medicaid-funded self-directed option. Nationally, about one third of eligible Medicaid HCBS recipients self-direct their services. The 2016 National Inventory reports 1,058,889 individuals self-directing in 253 programs (The National Resource Center for Participant-Directed Services, 2017).

But, why is the self-direction model especially helpful during this COVID-19 emergency? In addition to the shortage of other options, there are three major reasons:

(1) People with preexisting conditions want to limit the number of people in and out of their homes to reduce their exposure to COVID-19. Agency workers often see several clients and turnover frequently.
(2) Close family and friends, many of whom live with or near individuals with disabilities and already provide unpaid care, may be newly unemployed. By paying family caregivers, recipients are able to compensate those close to them instead of worrying that the care is an added burden. Research has shown that receiving assistance from people that the individual with disabilities already knows is beneficial (Newcomer et al., 2012). Conversely, family members experience less stress because they do not have to worry about the adequacy of care (Foster et al., 2007).
(3) Self-direction provides significant flexibility. The individual with disabilities can switch between agency-delivered and self-directed services at any time. When the program participant has control of the budget, (s)he can purchase needed goods and services including personal protective equipment (PPE), a cellphone, or internet connection to facilitate telehealth.

Recognizing that alternatives were needed, CMS released a toolkit to respond to the COVID-19 pandemic and increase access to alternatives to care in congregate settings. The Appendix K template, which helps states expedite changes to their 1915(c) home and community-based services waivers, explicitly permits states to request expansion of self-direction. Many of the same changes can be made to state plan-funded services using Section 1135.

Below are some highlights of what states have done in the first month after the CMS Toolkit was released to expand self-direction options under Appendix K.

Hiring legally responsible relatives

During the COVID-19 crisis, hiring legally responsible relatives (for example, a spouse or parent of a child with a disability) has become one of the most popular modifications requested. As of April 23, fourteen states have modified their waiver programs to permit the temporary hiring of legally responsible relatives, thus expanding the labor market significantly.

Increasing rates and budgets

Twenty-one states are increasing self-directed budgets, benefit limits, and/or rates.

Implementing other strategies

North Carolina is increasing budget limits by over 800 USD to allow more supplies and equipment to be purchased. Many states have added PPE to the list of permissible purchases. Colorado and New Jersey have increased individual budget limits to permit additional overtime. West Virginia is working with hospital discharge planners to bypass nursing home placements and enroll individuals directly into HCBS. Florida added personal supports and transportation to those services that may be self-directed.

Nearly half of all states use managed care plans to administer Medicaid HCBS. States typically require managed care plans to offer self-direction to their enrollees. New Jersey's State Plan 1115 waiver where 18,000 people are enrolled is a good example. Participants can spend up to 10% of their budgets for goods and services and a small amount of the budget can even be paid in cash.

Other changes allowed under the CMS toolkit are making the option more accessible; streamlining operations allowing (re)assessments and monitoring by phone, electronic signatures, timesheets submitted by phone, and temporarily waiving background checks and fingerprinting (which may be less necessary when hiring close family and friends).

The COVID-19 pandemic serves as a natural experiment. CMS and states have temporarily suspended various requirements which are meant to ensure safety and quality, but also slow, and in some cases seriously impede, timely access to HCBS. The pandemic offers an opportunity to reassess some of these requirements and ask whether they are really useful or might be modified once the immediate crisis is over. Benefits such as sick leave and health insurance coverage may become more widely available for personal care workers. If so, these jobs would become more attractive, easing the long-term worker shortage.

The data presented here are only for the first month when emergency provisions were in place. It will be interesting to measure changes in the delivery system over time. Perhaps change will occur due to societal values and preferences, and not just because of regulatory changes. How long will it be before people are comfortable placing a relative in a nursing facility? How long will close family, who are now able to provide additional care, be without other jobs? Will some family stay on as paid providers? Previous research suggests the answer is "Yes" (Benjamin et al., 2008).

Anthony Fauci, M.D. and other scientific experts have warned that the U.S. may never entirely return to "normal". At first this may seem ominous, but need not be so. If we reflect back in time, it was the polio epidemic that led to the self-direction movement as the people affected by that disease fought for greater control over their lives (Shapiro, 1994). Just as crises in the past have spurred new ways of thinking, COVID-19 may be opening our eyes anew to the value of self-direction. Who knows what the new "normal" will be?

Acknowledgement

The author would like to thank Suzanne Crisp, Molly Hurt Morris and Casey DeLuca for their assistance with the research and editing of this Commentary.

References

Benjamin, A. E., Matthias, R. E., Kathryn, K., & Furman, W. (2008). Retention of paid related caregivers: Who stays and who leaves home care careers? *The Gerontologist*, *48*(1, 1), 104–113. https://doi.org/10.1093/geront/48.Supplement_1.104

Carlson, B. L., Foster, L., Dale, S., & Brown, R. (2007). Effects of cash and counseling on personal care and well-being. *Health Services Research*, *42*(1 Pt 2), 467–487. https://doi.org/10.1111/j.1475-6773.2006.00673.x

Dolan, J., & Hamilton, M. (2020, April 7). *Consider pulling residents from nursing homes over coronavirus, says county health director*. Los Angeles Times Communications, LLC (Nant Capital): Los Angeles Times. https://www.latimes.com/california/story/2020-04-07/corona virus-nursing-homes-residents-remove-la-county

Foster, L., Dale, S. B., & Brown, R. (2007). How caregivers and workers fared in cash and counseling. *Health Services Research*, *42*(1 Pt 2), 510–532. https://doi.org/10.1111/j.1475-6773.2006.00672

The National Resource Center for Participant-Directed Services. (2017). *Publicly funded self-directed long-term services and supports programs in the United States*. AARP.

Newcomer, R. J., Kang, T., & Doty, P. (2012). Allowing spouses to be paid personal care providers: Spouse availability and effects on Medicaid-funded service use and expenditures. *The Gerontologist*, *52*(4), 517–530. https://doi.org/10.1093/geront/gnr102

Shapiro, J. P. (1994). *No pity: People with disabilities forging a new civil rights movement*. Broadway Books.

COVID-19 Pandemic: Opportunity to Advanced Home Care for Older Adults

Dear Editor,

A fundamental principle of geriatric care is to identify functional impairment and maximize residual function. During the COVID-19 pandemic, most of the developing and developed countries are ignorant of geriatric health needs. Therefore, a robust approach is highly essential that requires an integrated preparedness by addressing geriatric care (Mazumder et al., 2020). This pandemic around the world disproportionately impacts older adults, and we need to be cautious about the narrative linking this to older people (Applegate & Ouslander, 2020). The majority of older adults are using healthcare services, but during the current crisis, they have to self-isolate for a very long time (Armitage & Nellums, 2020).

Isolation among older adults is a "serious public health concern" because of their high risk for loneliness and other health problems. It might reduce transmission and minimize the spread to these high-risk groups, but if health sectors instruct older adults to remain home, they must have vital medical and home care and medications delivered (Armitage & Nellums, 2020). The healthcare team must be cognizant of the fact that each person experiences loneliness and social isolation in their own unique way, and our responses must be tailored to meet those individual needs and grounded in evidence-based practice in their homes (Berg-Weger & Morley, 2020). Thus, during this pandemic, policymakers have to seek health approaches to respond to some of these demands. This challenging situation is an unrepeatable opportunity for the development of home care services for older adults that is one of the most critical aspects of the elderly care and service program.

The shifting landscape of care, from formal – such as hospitals and rehabilitation services – to informal settings, including home, also influences the understanding of home as a place of care by older adults. Informal care is recognized as a significant resource in the care of older adults living with a chronic life-limiting illness (Compton et al., 2019). Coming to an understanding of growing older at home is essential because the entry of care providers redefines home as a caringscapes (Bowlby, 2012).

There is a need for increased knowledge and information about care and follow-up from home care services. Family caregivers are essential for promoting sustainable use, but a support system and better cooperation with home care services are needed (Karlsen et al., 2019). However, there is also call for more support with mastering particular skills and dealing with challenging situations. Due to the limitations of the COVID-19 pandemic, home health technologies could be to develop, and online technologies may provide health care at home. The use of telecare can reduce older adults' need for hospital admission, residential care, or other public care services and enable them to live for a longer time in their own homes. Future research is needed to understand better the factors that contribute to health care technology acceptance for older adults in general the same as it has been in the current crisis.

Vahidreza Borhaninejad

ⓘ http://orcid.org/0000-0002-4689-6741

Vahid Rashedi

ⓘ http://orcid.org/0000-0002-3972-3789

Disclosure statement

No financial interest or benefit has arisen from writing this paper.

References

Applegate, W. B., & Ouslander, J. G. (2020). COVID-19 presents high risk to older persons. *Journal of the American Geriatrics Society*, 68(4), 681. https://doi.org/10.1111/jgs.16426

Armitage, R., & Nellums, L. B. (2020). COVID-19 and the consequences of isolating the elderly. *The Lancet Public Health*, 5(5), e256. https://doi.org/10.1016/S2468-2667(20)30061-X

Berg-Weger, M., & Morley, J. E. (2020). Loneliness and social isolation in older adults during the covid-19 pandemic: implications for gerontological social work. *The Journal of Nutrition, Health & Aging*, 24(5), 456–458. https://doi.org/10.1007/s12603-020-1366-8

Bowlby, S. (2012). Recognising the time—space dimensions of care: Caringscapes and carescapes. *Environment & Planning A*, 44(9), 2101–2118. https://doi.org/10.1068/a44492

Compton, R. M., Owilli, A. O., Caine, V., Berendonk, C., Jouan-Tapp, D., Sommerfeldt, S. (2019). Home first: exploring the impact of community-based home care for older adults and their family caregivers. *Canadian Journal on Aging/La Revue Canadienne Du Vieillissement*:1–11. https://doi.org/10.1017/S0714980819000461

Karlsen, C., Moe, C. E., Haraldstad, K., & Thygesen, E. (2019). Caring by telecare? A hermeneutic study of experiences among older adults and their family caregivers. *Journal of Clinical Nursing*, 28(78), 1300–1313. https://doi.org/10.1111/jocn.14744

Mazumder, H., Hossain, M. M., & Das, A. (2020). Geriatric care during public health emergencies: lessons learned from novel corona virus disease (COVID-19) Pandemic. *Journal of Gerontological Social Work*, 1–2. https://doi.org/10.1080/01634372.2020.1746723

The Need for Community Practice to Support Aging in Place during COVID-19

Dear Editor,

While the COVID-19 pandemic has been devastating to 1.4 million nursing home residents in the US, it also has threatened the well-being of 50 million older adults who are aging in their own homes and apartments outside of licensed care facilities (Scheckler, 2020). Because older adults are at greater risk of mortality and health complications from the virus (Garnier-Crussard et al., 2020), officials are encouraging people ages 65 and older, in particular, to continue to practice social distancing as shelter-in-place orders are relaxed. As a result, many older adults today face ongoing challenges in accessing health-care services, home- and community-based services, as well as opportunities to connect with their communities' social infrastructure and their own private networks of family members and friends (Morrow-Howell et al., 2020).

Much of the calls to action for gerontological social workers and other professionals in aging during this pandemic have focused on the provision of direct services for older adults, especially for those living in residential care settings (Miller & Lee, 2020; Sands et al., 2020). It is important to note that social workers also have an opportunity to serve as leaders in aging by embracing a professional identity as agents of change within local, geographic-based communities. Practice that is oriented to communities as the client system is especially important for facilitating intergroup, inter-organizational, and interpersonal processes to transform and improve systems that affect the health and well-being of individuals who are aging in place during the pandemic.

Resources and media content from advocacy and professional organizations in aging demonstrate the heightened relevance of community-level work during the pandemic. As an example, the AARP Livable Communities Program expanded its Community Challenge Grants program to offer seed funding for innovative, collaborative, community projects in response to older adults' needs arising from the pandemic, such as access to basic needs and opportunities for engagement (AARP, n. d.). Additionally, through its partnership with the National League of Cities, AARP is amplifying the work of community leaders by creating an online platform that features programs and partnerships to support older adults within local COVID-19 response efforts (COVID Older Adult Response Initiative, n.d.).

More widespread involvement of social workers in such efforts is essential for broadening the scope, strengthening the effectiveness, and deepening the comprehensiveness of community-level responses to the strengths and needs of older adults and caregivers during this pandemic (Santiago & Smith, 2020). Social workers bring competencies to community practice and aging through:

- Understanding culturally responsive approaches to engaging diverse subgroups of older adults in systems-level change;
- Orienting to intersections of ageism with other forms of oppression, as well as processes of life course cumulative dis/advantage, that impact health, quality of life, and participation as people age;
- Adopting strengths-based and intergenerational orientations that recognize the interdependencies and contributions of residents of all ages;
- Facilitating effective interdisciplinary teamwork involving stakeholders with potentially different priorities, leading values, and resource levels;
- Recognizing the importance of helping to empower diverse subgroups older adults as leaders of their own communities; and
- Skills to lead advocacy efforts toward equity in the context of heterogeneous and unequal experiences of aging in community.

Our own research on the development of age-friendly community initiatives (AFCIs) in New Jersey has provided insights on the importance of community practitioners with expertise in the field of aging. We have observed that AFCI leaders who had cultivated strong collaborative interorganizational relationships prior to COVID-19 have been well positioned to team up with others to more quickly and comprehensively respond to older adults in their communities when shelter-in-place orders were first introduced (Taub Foundation, n.d.). It is especially important that social workers with expertise in aging are involved in community-level responses to COVID-19 to facilitate equity in marginalized and underserved communities and to broaden the reach of community collaborations. This is particularly salient in the current climate in which issues of racial injustice and widespread calls for action toward systemic reform are especially prominent at the local, national, and global levels. Social workers have an opportunity to encourage others to speak and act in support of anti-racist practices and systems change as part of age-friendly community change and aging-focused community responses to COVID-19 (for an example, see https://conta.cc/2MNIDkS).

Although social work competencies in aging historically have focused more on micro-practice, there has been growing emphasis more recently on macro and community practice. For example, the Council on Social Work Education's Gero-Ed Center added a section on "Leadership in the Practice Environment of Aging" as part of a tool to assess social work practice behaviors in the field of aging. These competencies go beyond the management of aging services and programs by addressing skills such as leadership through advocacy; building and managing collaborations across disciplines; and engaging in public communication (CSWE, n.d.). The pandemic accentuates the importance of such skills in aging to lead communities for this historical moment, as well as for the decades to come.

Althea Pestine-Stevens

http://orcid.org/0000-0001-7255-1088

Emily A. Greenfield

References

AARP. (n.d.). *AARP community challenge 2020 examples of potential coronavirus projects.* https://www.aarp.org/content/dam/aarp/livable-communities/community-challenge/2020/Coronavirus%20Challenge%20Examples.pdf

COVID Older Adult Response Initiative. (n.d.). https://covid19.nlc.org/resources/covid-19-older-adult-response-initiative/

CSWE Gero-Ed Center. (n.d.). *Geriatric social work competency scale II with lifelong leadership skills: Social work practice behaviors in the field of aging.* https://www.pogoe.org/sites/default/files/GeriatricSocialWorkCompetencyScaleII%26LifelongLeadershipSkills.pdf

Garnier-Crussard, A., Forestier, E., Gilbert, T., & Krolak-Salmon, P. (2020). Novel coronavirus (COVID-19) epidemic: What are the risks for older patients? *Journal of the American Geriatrics Society, 68*(5), 939–940. https://doi.org/10.1111/jgs.16407

Miller, V. J., & Lee, H. (2020). Social work values in action during COVID-19. *Journal of Gerontological Social Work.* Advance online publication. https://doi.org/10.1080/01634372.2020.1769792

Morrow-Howell, N., Galucia, N., & Swinford, E. (2020). Recovering from the COVID-19 pandemic: A focus on older adults. *Journal of Aging & Social Policy, 32*(4–5), 526–535. https://doi.org/10.1080/08959420.2020.1759758

Sands, L. P., Albert, S. M., & Suitor, J. J. (2020). Understanding and addressing older adults' needs during COVID-19. *Innovation in Aging, 4*(3), 1-3. https://doi.org/10.1093/geroni/igaa019

Santiago, A. M., & Smith, R. J. (2020). Community practice, social action, and the politics of pandemics. *Journal of Community Practice, 28*(2), 89–99. https://doi.org/10.1080/10705422.2020.1763744

Scheckler, S. (2020, April 17). *When family can't care for older adults during COVID-19, who will?* https://www.jchs.harvard.edu/blog/when-family-cant-care-for-older-adults-during-covid-19-who-will/

Taub Foundation. (n.d.). *Age-friendly leaders join in COVID-19 response efforts.* http://taub foundation.org/age-friendly-blog/age-friendly-leaders-join-in-covid-19-response-efforts/

Covid-19 and Community Care in South Korea

Dear Editor,

In South Korea, the bulk of confirmed cases of COVID-19 are due to a cluster infection in the Shincheonji Church (41.0% of total cases), small cluster infections in the community (26.2%), and imported infections from foreign countries (12.2%; Korea Centers for Disease Control and Prevention [KCDC], 2020). Although adults 60 and older constitute only 24% of all cases, 93% of the total COVID-19 related deaths occurred among this older group. The mortality rate (deaths/the number of reported cases) was approximately 200 times higher for individuals in their eighties than for those in their thirties (KCDC, 2020). Older adults staying in long-term care institutions including nursing homes and long-term care hospitals are particularly vulnerable. Fourteen percent of 3,330 cases from small cluster infections were from long-term care institutions, and 54.6% of total deaths were related to care institutions and hospitals.

A shortage of qualified home-based care services in South Korea means that most older people have no choice but to depend heavily on residential institutional care. From 2012 to 2017, the number of long-term residential care facility beds per thousand people aged 65 years old and over significantly increased from 51.1 to 60.9, and the number of beds in long-term care hospitals was the 36.7 per thousand people, the highest among OECD countries (OECD, 2019).

Cost and preference are among the concerns people have raised regarding institutional care. For example, because residential institutional care is financially supported by the universally accessible national health insurance (NHI) and Long-Term Care Insurance (LTCI), lengthy hospitalizations in the long-term care hospital (187 days on average) can threaten the financial sustainability of the health system (Hwang et al., 2016). Moreover, a survey shows that more than 50% of older people desire to live independently in their own communities rather than in residential institutions (Jung et al., 2017). The spread of COVID-19 has raised more concerns about institutional care. The recent outbreak revealed that care institutions are particularly vulnerable to COVID-19 for the following reasons (Gardner et al., 2020; Lai et al., 2020): (a) the high population density of long term care hospitals (the number of beds in one room is 5.12 on average in long-term care hospitals while it is 3.61 in general hospitals), (b) difficulties in requiring people with dementia or respiratory disease to observe needed hygiene or wear masks; (c) the preexisting health conditions of most residents in care institutions that make them more susceptible to infection. With these ongoing problems of institutional care, there is a growing need for aging at home strategies.

In 2018, the Korean Government announced its "Community Care" policy initiative to shift the paradigm from institution-based to community-based care. Community Care aims to enhance the quality of life and overall well-being of the older adults by providing home care tailored to their needs (KMOHW, 2018). Furthermore, it aims to improve the financial sustainability of the NHI by reducing "social admission," referring to the admission of older people into hospitals for care services rather than for medical needs. Community Care has also now received attention from advocates and researchers who wish to reduce cluster infections during pandemics.

I recommend the following policy strategies to enable the shift toward home care. First, efforts should be made to keep older persons healthy at home as long as possible, for example, by collaborating with primary health-care providers such as doctors, nurses, and pharmacists to provide appropriate medical services (Jeon & Kwon, 2017). Next, given that the transmission risk is particularly high between people in close contact, it is necessary to employ technological aids and minimize face-to-face contact. Finally, considering the potential for outbreaks based in adult daycare centers, which offer social and recreation services for older adults staying in their own communities, these centers should require staff and users to adhere to hygiene rules such as washing hands thoroughly, wearing masks, and keeping distance from one another.

Soyoon Weon

ⓘ http://orcid.org/0000-0002-8633-9368

References

Gardner, W., States, D., & Bagley, N. (2020). The coronavirus and the risks to the elderly in long-term care. *Journal of Aging & Social Policy*, *32*(4–5), 310–315. https://doi.org/10.1080/08959420.2020.1750543

Hwang, D. K., Kim, T. W., Park, K. R., & Yeo, N. K. (2016). *Actual condition in long-term hospitalized patient receiving medical benefits (Policy report No. 2015–24)*. Korea Institute for Health and Social Affairs [KIHASA]. http://repository.kihasa.re.kr:8080/handle/201002/15352

Jeon, B., & Kwon, S. (2017). Health and long-term care systems for older people in the Republic of Korea: Policy challenges and lessons. *Health Systems & Reform*, *3*(3), 214–223. https://doi.org/10.1080/23288604.2017.1345052

Jung, K. H., Oh, Y. H., Kang, E. N., Kim, K. R., Lee, Y. K., Oh, M. A., Hwang, N. H., Kim, S. J., Lee, S. H., Lee, S. K., & Hong, S. Y. (2017). *A survey on the actual condition of the elderly in Korea (Policy report No. 2017)*. KIHASA. http://www.mohw.go.kr/react/jb/sjb030301vw.jsp?PAR_MENU_ID=03&MENU_ID=032901&page=1&CONT_SEQ=344953

KMOHW. (2020). *Number of hospital beds in South Korea, 2019* [Data set]. https://www.mohw.go.kr/react/gm/sgm0601vw.jsp?PAR_MENU_ID=13&MENU_ID=1304020303&page=1&CONT_SEQ=293339

Korea Centers for Disease Control and Prevention [KCDC]. (2020, June 28). *Cases and deaths in the South Korea.* https://www.cdc.go.kr/board/board.es?mid=a30402000000&bid=0030

Korean Ministry of Health and Welfare [KMOHW]. (2018, November 20). *Basic plan on the community care.* http://www.mohw.go.kr/react/al/sal0301vw.jsp?PAR_MENU_ID=04&MENU_ID=0403&page=2&CONT_SEQ=346683&SEARCHKEY=TITLE&SEARCHVALUE=%EB%8F%8C%EB%B4%84

Lai, -C.-C., Wang, J.-H., Ko, W.-C., Yen, M.-Y., Lu, M.-C., Lee, C.-M., & Hsueh, P.-R. (2020). COVID-19 in long-term care facilities: An upcoming threat that cannot be ignored. *Journal of Microbiology, Immunology, and Infection*, *53*(3), 444–446. https://doi.org/10.1016/j.jmii.2020.04.008

Organization for Economic Co-operation and Development [OECD]. (2019). *Health statistics, 2019* [Data set]. https://stats.oecd.org/Index.aspx?ThemeTreeId=9

Social Work with Older Persons Living with Dementia in Nigeria: COVID-19

Dear Editor,

The world's population is gradually aging. Dementia and other cognitive impairments are becoming a global health priority because of their increasing prevalence (World Health Organisation, 2019). In the Sub-Saharan African region, dementia has posed an impending crisis on older individuals. Globally, there are over 50 million people with dementia, with the presentation of new cases every 3 seconds (Alzheimer's Disease International, 2019). It has also been predicted that by 2050, there will be a 250% increase in the number of people with dementia. There are no existing nationally representative data about the prevalence of dementia in Nigeria, but there is 4.9% prevalence of dementia in Nigeria, with 6.7% high prevalence in women compared to men and common among older persons who are above 70 years (Ogunniyi et al., 2000)

The double attack of dementia and COVID-19 is a major concern for persons living with dementia and their family members. Given the novelty of the COVID-19 virus, how rapidly public health situation is evolving around the world, and the negative impact it has had on older persons with chronic health condition like dementia (World Health Organization, 2020), there is a need for appropriate psychosocial intervention tailored to individuals with dementia. Clinical presentation of patients who died as a result of COVID-19 showed comorbidities of hypertension and cardiac ischemic diseases; however, dementia was categorized as a comorbid health condition among 6.8% of COVID-19 patients in developed countries like Italy (Onder et al., 2020). Although dementia has been recognized as a risk factor among older persons who are above 60 years of age, there are no studies that explain the implication of dementia as a factor influencing the mortality of patients affected by COVID-19 around the world (D'Adamo et al., 2020).

Social service workers in Nigeria are essential in the provision of psycho-social support to older persons with dementia especially during this COVID-19 pandemic, by working with individuals and their family members. The Nigerian Government has been working to curtail the spread of the virus and its impact on the citizens. People are also trying to adhere to several preventive measures such as limiting contact with others, regular hand washing, maintaining social distancing, and self-isolation in a case where individuals have developed symptoms of the virus.

Compulsory social distance presents its challenges as older persons may struggle with isolation, limited access to health services, and restricted mobility which leads to poor access to financial resources. Most older persons in Nigeria reside in rural areas where social distancing might have a greater effect on them, especially those who are frail, who are very old, or with multiple chronic health conditions. However, these traits also make them highly susceptible to COVID-19 (Zhou et al., 2020). Because of aggressive physical distancing and changes in health-care delivery systems in the country, older persons with a chronic health condition like dementia may have adapted very poorly to the pandemic.

Since there is a paucity of information about the impact of COVID-19 on older persons with dementia, social workers are an essential workforce in providing care and psychosocial support. T his special group often has difficulty communicating their feelings and experience, and require extra vigilance in terms of observation and reporting any new and unusual activities (Rgptoronto.ca, 2020). Older persons with dementia during COVID-19 often have difficulty in processing messages, including safety procedures such as wearing of the mask including public health information (World Health Organization, 2020). This has resulted in feelings of frustrations, loneliness, and withdrawal from the social environment. The rights and care needs of older persons with dementia have not been fully recognized during the COVID-19 pandemic and may add to feeling stigmatized, isolated, and unable to participate in the public life of their communities (Brooker et al., 2014).

Caregivers of older persons with dementia may experience psychological strains as a result of lockdown (Prince et al., 2011; Thomas & Milli = gan, 2015). This period of social distancing has posed emotional and social stress to informal caregivers because formal caregiving agencies are closed down. Home-based caregivers are equally not allowed to move around to provide essential care services for older persons with dementia and other cognitive impairments during the COVID-19 pandemic. Older persons with dementia in nursing homes lost physical contact with their family members and activities when visits to Nigeria were prohibited. Most social workers working in the homes have become more isolated; they practice compassionate care under fear of infection and stress about the clinical condition of their patients. There have been signs of exhaustion and burnout during the period of lockdown in all facilities.

Therefore, identifying the care needs of older persons with dementia during pandemics like COVID-19 is important. Social workers are identified as frontline essential workers with care needs. The British Association of Social Workers has developed guidance for them to look after themselves by not neglecting sick days and taking days off to rest, maintaining personal routines like physical exercise, speaking to friends, and getting good sleep. As services become overwhelmed during the pandemic, social workers need to know their limits and learn when to say 'no,' they must be able to identify clear support systems (professionally and personally), be able to ask questions when uncertain about things, try to limit their exposure to news updates on social media, seek supervision, and try to use appropriate humor in a supportive context during the pandemic (British Association of Social Workers, 2020).

A well-supported and appropriately equipped social worker is essential for reducing the damaging impact of the COVID-19 pandemic on older persons with dementia in Nigeria. It is also imperative for government and non-government organizations to redress the pending social needs of older persons with dementia such as the provision of psychosocial support delivered by social workers including meditation exercise delivered through electronic platforms and behavioral management supported through the telephone hotlines. Distress helplines can be established to serve older persons with dementia experiencing abuse. Individuals with parents that have dementia are encouraged to spend more time with them by taking up some caregiving duties while professional carers get some respite time for themselves. Meeting the care needs of older persons with dementia during the pandemic is an integral part of the fulfillment of fundamental human rights of the new United Nations Convention.

Oluwagbemiga Oyinlola

Oluromade Olusa

References

Alzheimer's Disease International. (2018) *Dementia World Alzheimer's report 2019: Attitudes to dementia. September, 2019.* Retrieved from https://www.alz co.uk/research/WorldAlzheimerReport2019. pdf

Alzheimer's Disease International. (2019). *World Alzheimer's report 2019: Attitudes to dementia.* https://www.alz.co.uk/research/WorldAlzheimerReport2019.pdf

Alzheimer's Disease International. (2020). *ADI offers advice and support during COVID-19.* 73rd World Health Assembly Statement submitted by Alzheimer's Disease International. Alzheimer's Disease International. London. UK. https://www.alz.co.uk/news/adi-offers-advice-and-support-during-covid-19.

British Association of Social Workers. (2020). *Quick guide: Self-care for social workers during COVID-19.* https://www.basw.co.uk/quick-guide-self-care-social-workers-during-covid-19

Brooker, D., La Fontaine, J., Evans, S., & Saad, K. (2014). Public health guidance to facilitate timely diagnosis of dementia: Alzheimer's Cooperative valuation in Europe recommendations. *International Journal of Geriatric Psychiatry, 29*(7), 682–693. https://doi.org/10.1002/gps.4066

D'Adamo, H., Yoshikawa, T., & Ouslander, J. G. (2020). Coronavirus disease 2019 in geriatrics and long-term care: The ABCDs of COVID-19. *Journal of the American Geriatrics Society, 68* (5), 912-917. https://doi.org/10.1111/jgs.1644

Ogunniyi, A., Baiyewu, O., Gureje, O., Hall, K. S., Unverzagt, F., Siu, S. H., Gao, S., Farlow, M., Oluwole, O. S. A., Komolafe, O., & Hendrie, H. C. (2000). Epidemiology of dementia in Nigeria: Results from the Indianapolis-Ibadan study. *European Journal of Neurology, 7*(5), 485–490. https://doi.org/10.1046/j.1468-1331.2000.00124.x

Onder, G., Rezza, G., & Brusaferro, S. (2020). Case-fatality rate and characteristics of patients dying in relation to COVID-19 in Italy. *JAMA - Journal of the American Medical Association, 323*(18), 1775-1776. https://doi.org/10.1001/jama.2020.468

Prince, M., Bryce, R., & Ferri, C. (2011). *Alzheimer's disease international—World Alzheimer report 2011: The benefits of early diagnosis and intervention.* Alzheimer's Disease International, UK. Retrievde from http://www.alz.co.uk/research/WorldAlzheimerReport2011.pdf

Rgptoronto.ca. 2020. *COVID-19 in older adults.* [online]. Regional Geriatric Program of Toronto, Canada. Retrieved from https://www.rgptoronto.ca/wp-content/uploads/2020/04/COVID-19-Presentations-in-Frail-Older-Adults-U-of-C-and-U-fo-T.pdf

Thomas, C., & Milli=gan, C. (2015). *How can and should UK society adjust to dementia?* Joseph Rowntree Foundation. Retrieved from http://www.jrf.org.uk/publications/how-can-and-should-uk-society-adjust-dementia

World Health Organisation. (2019). *Coronavirus disease 2019 (COVID-19) situation report-79.* World Health Organisation, Geneva, Switzerland. Retrieved from http://www.who.int/docs/default-source/coronavirus/situation-report/202000498-sitrep-79-covid-19.pdf?sfvrsn=4796b1443_4

World Health Organization. 2020. https://www.who.int/emergencies/diseases/novelcorona virus- 2019/situation-reports/.

Zhou, F., Yu, T., Du, R., Fan, G., Liu, Y., Liu, Z., Xiang, J., Wang, Y., Song, B., Gu, X., Guan, L., Wei, Y., Li, H., Wu, X., Xu, J., Tu, S., Zhang, Y., Chen, H., & Cao, B. (2020). Clinical course and risk factors for mortality of adult inpatients with COVID-19 in Wuhan, China: A retrospective cohort study. *The Lancet, 395*(10229), 1054–1062. https://doi.org/10.1016/S0140-6736(20)30566-3

Thoughts on Living in a Nursing Facility during the Pandemic

Dear Editor,

As a nursing home resident and nursing home advocate, it is with dread that I now read the Boston Globe and open my inbox each morning to read the latest updates about how the COVID-19 pandemic is affecting us.

I am especially horrified by the devastation that the coronavirus contagion is causing inside American nursing facilities as in New Jersey where 17 bodies piled up, and about the large number of residents in a Seattle one that perished. Here in Massachusetts, 1700 residents of long-term care facilities have died, 76 in a single facility – the Soldiers' Home in Holyoke.

I personally have been living in a nursing facility for 18 years due to functional limitations from an acute episode of Guillain-Barre syndrome. I have quadraparesis – weakness in all four limbs. I cannot walk. I am total care. I need to be washed, dressed and transferred to my power chair.

The facility in which I live is not typical. In most facilities, residents are described primarily as elderly frail people over 80, often with underlying health conditions. These older individuals are at the highest risk to COVID-19 as it is so contagious. But our population is different – receiving specialized care mostly for neurological and psychiatric disorders. Our residents are generally younger – ages 21–65. They are still at risk.

In my facility we have COVID-positive residents and our management has responded to the pandemic by following CMS' guidance with preventative measures. We bar visitors, implement social distancing, have eliminated congregate dining, screen staff daily and provide staff with personal protective equipment – plastic face shields, masks, gowns, gloves and sanitizer – as precautions to avoid transmission of the virus.

I find my facility very changed. I am now acutely aware of the number of people I encounter in our crowded halls, the difficulty of physically distancing ourselves in a congregate living and working environment.

I see staff wearing their protective equipment, and not seeing some staff who are missing as they are fearful and staying home. I am alarmed when I hear that there's an emergency, a resident who's having trouble breathing and needs to be sent out to a hospital. I am troubled that three residents on my unit have died, not knowing whether they died of the virus or not. I am distressed to find of the two nursing assistants getting me up one morning one is the cousin of a nursing assistant in another facility who died of the virus, and whose death was the subject of an article in the Boston Globe.

Although I realize that our staff are anxious, stressed and understaffed, heroic for even coming to work which puts them at risk for their health and lives, I still expect that they will provide crisis standards of care.

I am frightened when they don't, especially when I see staff not following basic infection control practices – a nursing assistant letting a resident who touches the ice in our ice chest get ice, a member of our Rehab staff putting my roommate's dirty linen on my overbed table and on my bookcase on top of my linen and personal papers. Staff not changing their gloves between touching different residents. I have heard multiple facility-wide pages from our central kitchen staff pleading for direct-care staff to not put their dirty gloves on trays being sent back to the kitchen after meals.

Even a COVID-positive resident who was not properly quarantined came into my room.

I believe that our performance would be better if our owner – who made a profit on our facility of over 2 USD million dollars in fiscal 2018 – provided us with more money to incentivize staff to come to work. We could do better also, if all staff followed basic infection control practices more vigilantly, rather than being lax which I have detailed they are not all doing.

I have to confront psychological effects and emotional challenges as I am feeling vulnerable. I have a sense of urgency about my life. I am fearful because such a large percentage of those dying were living in LTC facilities and I am living with those who have the virus. I think often of my mortality, wondering if I will succumb to this pandemic, whether this will be the time for me to leave our planet. Should I be writing goodbye letters to significant people in my life thanking them for their contributions to my life? This thinking about my mortality is not easy.

What can we learn from this unexpected crisis about people with disabilities living in nursing homes? I feel strongly that the money for long-term care reimbursements should be put into the hands of individuals and families to give us the choice of where to get needed services and supports. The importance of having the choice to be able to receive home and community-based services, to be included in the community has been high-lighted by the dangerousness of living in crowded institutions during a contagious pandemic.

Disturbingly, this choice is impossible for me personally as MassHealth's -the Massachusetts Medicaid program – current policy regarding the extent of community-based services I am eligible for is insufficient for me to live outside an institution. Everyone – even me who requires a lot of care – should have the right to control where and how to receive needed care and supports.

The extraordinary number of individuals who have contacted COVID-19 in long-term care facilities and have died underscores the urgency of reforming our long-term care support system to eliminate the inequities by giving those of us with disabilities the option to receive more humane safer care in the community.

Sincerely,

Penny Shaw

The Care Home Pandemic – What Lessons Can We Learn for the Future?

Dear Editor,

Whilst the world is still getting to grips with the impact of COVID-19, another crisis slowly emerges in care homes across the world. Older adults have already been identified as vulnerable to the devastation of COVID –19, but death rates in care homes have risen exponentially with tragic stories being heard from across the world in recent days.

Case fatality rates for countries with older populations have been damning, with over 95% of deaths in these populations in those over the age of 60 (Kluge, 2020). In the UK, deaths from all causes in care homes have increased by over 200% since the start of the outbreak (Foundation, 2020). Governments have correctly identified that the geriatric population need protection in pandemics such as the one we currently find ourselves in. Mortality rates are higher in those patients with comorbidities, especially with the added risk of comorbidities being present in these elder age groups (Guan et al., 2020). This begs the question as to why those in care homes have been left so helpless?

Analyzing a study of the COVID-19 outbreak in an American care-home showed the contagiosity of this coronavirus, with over 60% of the residents reporting as positive for the virus (Gardner et al., 2020). Across Europe, traumatic stories from care workers continued to sieve through and a running theme emerged of unanswered pleas for extra support to put a stop to this silent massacre. Heartening accounts have been rare but one care home in Lyon, France took the decision for staff to isolate with residents in the care home in a determined effort to save their residents, several weeks later all the staff tested negative for the virus (Gauriat, 2020).

Even in times of crisis, social workers and other staff members continue to serve on the frontline and provide services to vulnerable older adults. Effective measures need to be implemented in a uniform manner to help better protect care home residents and their staff. The sparsity of resources available for staff needs to be addressed with the provision and access to adequate personal protective equipment being made early. Following WHO hand hygiene models along with sanitizer provision can help reduce the spread of the infection (Mona Koshkouei & Pilbeam, 2020). Along with this efficient management of staff and their allocation in care homes is needed to avoid excessive movement of staff as they can become potential entry points for the virus. Similarly, visitors need to be told to stay away to help protect their loved ones from excessive exposure. Rapid access to efficient testing and detection of cases can help minimize the spread of the virus in these settings and in the long haul save the lives of these vulnerable adults (Mona Koshkouei & Pilbeam, 2020).

These adaptations are no easy feat, but with health-care systems buckling under the high demands in these unprecedented times, any lessons learned now could be crucial to prevent such tragedies from reoccurring.

Ameer A. Khan

ⓘ http://orcid.org/0000-0001-
8768-6209

Vineshwar P. Singh and Darab Khan

References

Gardner, W., States, D., & Bagley, N. (2020, April 3). The Coronavirus and the risks to the elderly in long-term care. *Journal of Aging & Social Policy*, *32*(4-5), 1–6. https://doi.org/10.1080/08959420.2020.1750543

Gauriat, V. (2020). *The deadly impact of Covid-19 on Europe's care homes*. euronews. Retrieved May 12, 2020, from https://www.euronews.com/2020/05/08/the-deadly-impact-of-covid-19-on-europe-s-care-home

Guan, W.-J., Liang, W.-H., Zhao, Y., Liang, H.-R., Chen, Z.-S., Li, Y.-M., Liu, X.-Q., Chen, R.-C., Tang, C.-L., Wang, T., Ou, C.-Q., Li, L., Chen, P.-Y., Sang, L., Wang, W., Li, J.-F., Li, -C.-C., Ou, L.-M., Cheng, B., Xiong, S., . . . China Medical Treatment Expert Group For, C. (2020). Comorbidity and its impact on 1590 patients with Covid-19 in China: A nationwide analysis. *The European respiratory journal*, *55*(5), 2000547. https://doi.org/10.1183/13993003.00547-2020

Kluge, D. H. H. P. (2020). *Statement – Older people are at highest risk from COVID-19, but all must act to prevent community spread*. World Health Organization(WHO)/Europe. Retrieved May 12, 2020, from http://www.euro.who.int/en/health-topics/health-emergencies/coronavirus-covid-19/statements/statement-older-people-are-at-highest-risk-from-covid-19,-but-all-must-act-to-prevent-community-spread

Mona Koshkouei, L. A., & Pilbeam, C. (2020). *How can pandemic spreads be contained in care homes?* CEBM (The Centre for Evidence Based Medicine). Retrieved May 12, 2020, from https://www.cebm.net/covid-19/how-can-pandemic-spreads-be-contained-in-care-homes/

The Health Foundation. (2020). *Care homes have seen the biggest increase in deaths since the start of the outbreak*. Retrieved May 12, 2020, from https://www.health.org.uk/news-and-comment/charts-and-infographics/deaths-from-any-cause-in-care-homes-have-increased

Nursing Home in the COVID-19 Outbreak: Challenge, Recovery, and Resiliency

Dear Editor,

A group of novel cases of viral pneumonia was first reported in Wuhan City, Hubei Province, on December 31, 2019, after which the disease spread rapidly around the world. On January 30, the World Health Organization (WHO) recognized the growing number of cases as a Public Health Emergency of International Concern (PHEIC) (Word Health Organization, 2005), and officially named it "COVID-19" on February 11th (Word Health Organization, 2020). COVID-19 now poses a great challenge to global public health, one of its tragedies being the disproportionate number of deaths among older adults. In China, as of February 11, 2020, people older than 60 years accounted for only 31.13% of the confirmed cases but 81.04% of the deaths attributed to COVID-19 (Team TNCPERE, 2020).

Compared with other nursing clinical practices, the nursing home (NH) sector received less attention and was slower to respond to this pandemic, with the most painful consequences (Fallon et al., 2020). An earlier study related to NHs revealed that 85.59% of residents contracted the disease (McMichael et al., 2020). Age is an important factor of poor prognosis of COVID-19 (Zhou et al., 2020). Weakness, dysfunction, cognitive impairment, malnutrition, multiple complications, and gregariousness increase the susceptibility of old-age residents (Etard et al., 2020). In addition, a sense of crisis was poorly perceived among this population as there were no atypical symptoms that would indicate an unusual cause of death.

However, from another perspective, the pandemic has further exposed the lack of experience and resources for NHs to respond to Public Health Emergencies (PHE). In fact, during other outbreaks of infectious disease including SARS in 2003, H1N1 influenza virus in 2009, H7N9 bird flu in 2013, Middle East Respiratory Syndrome (MERS) in 2015, Ebola in 2018, and COVID-19 in 2020, densely populated settlements of older individuals at not only NHs but also long-term care institutions such as skilled nursing and assisted living institutions, have always been the most vulnerable. At this stage, it is time for us to seriously reflect on how to ensure that NHs can respond to and survive disasters, stress, or changes of the environment, that is, how to enhance our resilience to future health threats.

Resilience is defined as the ability to quickly recover to an original state after suffering from external forces (Tompkins & Hurlston-McKenzie, 2011). It is generally believed that when an emergency occurs, a resilient organization can feed back useful information and urge the government to make decisions, so as to cooperate or partner with the government. Qinggang nursing home, China's first nursing home approved by the national development and reform commission, was set up by a first-class tertiary hospital, as the vanguard and pilot base of a nursing care institution in China, becoming famous throughout the country for its integration of medical care and nursing. We declared a "state of alert" and adopted a series of resilient strategies when the COVID-19 pandemic was first declared and achieved "zero infection" among 335 residents and 276 health-care personnel. The following are some general strategies that can be used for reference:

- Emergency management
  - Launch public health emergency plans and establish an emergency management team and formulate and implement the emergency response plan for COVID-19 prevention and control in nursing institutions.
  - Establish quarantine sections by dividing space into living quarters, work stations, and staff living quarters, and set up a buffer room between two passageways and three zones. The boundaries between the districts should be clear and obvious.
  - Release a formal notice of quarantine and obtain the understanding and cooperation of the older adults and their families. Close all entrances and exits of the organization, leaving only one passageway in and out. Set up a receiving and testing point for external drugs, express parcels, and vehicles, adjusted to meet local government and quarantine requirements as well as allow families to make an appointment for ordered visitation.
- Staff management and training
  - Comprehensively screen epidemiological history and track activity and physical health status of employees in the two weeks before commencing employment, implement closed management, and rotate every 14 days.
  - Give priority to online training for all personnel in the organization, especially non-front-line staff such as security, cleaning, greening, catering, etc. The training contents include but are not limited to basic knowledge regarding COVID-19, hand hygiene, mask wearing, disinfection, isolation, etc.
  - During the quarantine, managers should be mindful that the increase of workload, worries about families, and own safety require the organization to identify employees' negative emotions and provide support, such as humanistic scheduling, mindfulness training, or psychological counseling.
- Care of older adults
  - Enhance basic caring for the disabled and semi-disabled older adults and pay attention to the observation and treatment of chronic diseases

such as hypertension, diabetes, coronary heart disease, and so on. Caregiver is responsible for monitoring and reporting the situation of the older adults at a fixed time on a daily basis.

o Highlight psychological support, provide information and scientific knowledge on the pandemic through official channels in the form of videos and health brochures, and assess cognitive, emotional, and behavioral changes in the older adults to provide help and support.

o Patients suspected of having COVID-19 should be isolated in a single room immediately to avoid close contact. At the same time, cases should be reported to local community health agencies and disease control agencies. Assist in the personal protection of the older adults and employees during the process of referrals.

As the global population ages and the life expectancy grows, increased growth in the demand for aged-care services of nursing homes is predicted. We suggest that nursing homes in all countries should learn from this tragedy and increase their capacity to help older adults, health-care workers, care-givers, and managers withstand this current pandemic, as well as the next unforeseen disaster.

Huanhuan Huang

 http://orcid.org/0000-0003-0845-7526
Yan Xie

Zhiyu Chen

Mingzhao Xiao

Songmei Cao

Jie Mi

Xiuli Yu

Qinghua Zhao

Acknowledgments

We acknowledged all the colleagues combating COVID-19.

Funding

This study was funded by Key Projects of Chongqing Science and Technology Commission foundation (cstc2018jscx-maszdX00113) and COVID-19 Emergency Clinical Research Project of Chongqing Medical University (2020-13-19).

Conflict of interest

The authors have no relevant financial information or potential conflicts to disclose.

Authors' contribution

HH H and Y X: conception, literature search, writing, major revision, and final approval.
ZY C: major revision, data collection, and final approval.
MZ X: conception, major revision, and final approval
SM C, J M and XL Y: editing, major revision, and final approval
QH Z: conception, supervision, major revision, and final approval

References

Etard, J.-F., Vanhems, P., Atlani-Duault, L., & Ecochard, R. (2020). Potential lethal outbreak of coronavirus disease (COVID-19) among the elderly in retirement homes and long-term facilities, France, March 2020. *Eurosurveillance*, 25(15), 2000448. https://doi.org/10.2807/1560-7917.ES.2020.25.15.2000448

Fallon, A., Dukelow, T., Kennelly, S. P., & O'Neill, D. (2020). COVID-19 in nursing homes. QJM: An International Journal of Medicine, 113(6),391–392. from https://doi.org/10.1093/qjmed/hcaa136

McMichael, T. M., Currie, D. W., Clark, S., Pogosjans, S., Kay, M., Schwartz, N. G., Lewis, J., Baer, A., Kawakami, V., Lukoff, M. D., Ferro, J., Brostrom-Smith, C., Rea, T. D., Sayre, M. R., Riedo, F. X., Russell, D., Hiatt, B., Montgomery, P., Rao, A. K., Chow, E. J., . . . Public Health–Seattle and King County, EvergreenHealth, and CDC COVID-19 Investigation Team (2020). Epidemiology of Covid-19 in a long-term care facility in King county, Washington. The New

England journal of medicine, 382(21),2005–2011. from https://doi.org/10.1056/NEJMoa2005412

Team TNCPERE. (2020). The epidemiological characteristics of an outbreak of 2019 novel coronavirus diseases (COVID-19) in China. *Chinese Journal of Epidemiology*, *41*(2), 145–151. from https://doi.org/10.3760/cma.j..0254-6450.2020.02.003

Tompkins, E., & Hurlston-McKenzie, L.-A. (2011). Public-private partnerships in the provision of environmental governance: A case of disaster management. In E. Boyd & C. Folke Eds., *Adapting institutions: Governance, complexity and social-ecological resilience* (pp. 171–189). Cambridge University Press. Retrieved May 9, 2020, from https://eprints.soton.ac.uk/202835/

Word Health Organization. (2005). *Statement on the second meeting of the international health regulations (2005) emergency committee regarding the outbreak of novel coronavirus (2019-nCoV)*. Published January 30, 2020. Retrieved April 30, 2020, from https://www.who.int/news-room/detail/30-01-2020-statement-on-the-second-meeting-of-the-international-health-regulations-(2005)-emergency-committee-regarding-the-outbreak-of-novel-coronavirus-(2019-ncov)

Word Health Organization. (2020). *WHO director-general's remarks at the media briefing on 2019-nCoV on 11 February 2020*. Published February 11, 2020. Retrieved April 30, 2020, from https://www.who.int/dg/speeches/detail/who-director-general-s-remarks-at-the-media-briefing-on-2019-ncov-on-11-february-2020

Zhou, F., Yu, T., Du, R., Fan, G., Liu, Y., Liu, Z., Xiang, J., Wang, Y., Song, B., Gu, X. and Guan, L. (2020). Clinical course and risk factors for mortality of adult inpatients with COVID-19 in Wuhan, China: A retrospective cohort study. *Lancet*, *395*(10229), 1054–1106. from https://doi.org/10.1016/S0140-6736(20)30566-3

Nursing Home Social Work During COVID-19

Dear Editor,

As the impacts of COVID-19 on nursing facilities became apparent, the members of the U.S. based National Nursing Home Social Work Network (NNHSWN) immediately considered what it could offer as a useful response to assist nursing home social workers working in facilities. The NNHSWN was brought together nearly a decade ago by Dr. Mercedes Bern-Klug at the University of Iowa School of Social Work and Bob Connolly, a social worker and Centers for Medicare and Medicaid Services (CMS) retiree who had worked on developing the Minimum Data Set or MDS. Membership consists primarily of social work researchers interested in nursing homes, most of whom have work experience in that setting. Readers of this journal may be familiar with Dr. Bern-Klug's and Mr. Connolly's publication and work on obtaining comments and policy suggestions on the proposed nursing home regulations in 2016 (Bern-Klug et al., 2016).

During some initial organizing calls that included a social work director at a nursing home in a hard-hit area, it became clear that COVID-19 presented many challenges for social services staff in nursing homes. For instance, social workers and nursing homes needed to figure out effective ways to communicate with family members. Some basic steps, like obtaining the e-mail addresses for family members, were not standard in some facilities and those who waited until their nursing home had a COVID-19 outbreak found it too late to initiate such protocols. Often, social workers found themselves making calls to update family members who were stressed, frightened, and frustrated.

When visitation restrictions were implemented, many social workers were also involved in helping residents stay connected to their families. This task proved to be challenging as access to technology was sporadic, and access to personal protective equipment (PPE), even worse. With PPE shortages nationally and nursing homes not being prioritized for PPE, many social workers were unable to obtain PPE, as it was reserved for the "frontline workers". Lack of PPE hampered social workers' ability to assist with communication. One social service director warned her administrator not to overpromise what the facility could provide in regards to video calls and other regular communication. Between mounting cases of COVID-19 and shortages of PPE, the ability to assist residents with video calls and maintain regular communication declined over time.

Social workers also faced ethical dilemmas, existential crises, stress, and fears. They were thrust into having difficult conversations about advance directives with the family members of very ill patients over the phone. Some social workers were labeled "non-essential" and asked to work from home or to avoid care units. How does one provide counseling and psychosocial care when one cannot access the resident directly? Nursing home social workers had to figure out how to conduct their work remotely with frail residents, some of whom already had communication challenges. Like many other nursing home workers, their workload increased dramatically with additional tasks. Also like other nursing home workers, many feared contracting COVID-19 and bringing it home to their families. In some cases, their families feared for them and did not understand why they continued to work in nursing homes at a risk to their own health.

We realized there were actions the NNHSWN could take to address these challenges. Guided by our original question of, "What we can do to help?", we did three things. First, we took our existing nursing home social work resource page https://clas.uiowa.edu/socialwork/nursing-home/national-nursing-home -social-work-network (University of Iowa School of Social Work, n.d.) and updated it with a cultivated list of resources to help nursing home social workers with the new responsibilities of their jobs. In subgroups, we combed the vast resources that were being generated almost on a daily basis and posted links to those we felt were the most succinct, the most accurate, and the most relevant. Second, we created weekly, then bi-weekly, online resilience-building support sessions via Zoom for those working in nursing homes. These sessions, facilitated by members of the NNHSWN and other research colleagues, provided a space for people in social service roles in nursing homes to hear from others with similar challenges, and to take time for themselves to de-stress, process trauma, and find solutions to the dilemmas presented to them on a daily basis. Finally, the NNHSWN disseminated information about the updated website and the support sessions through a nursing home social work listserv also hosted through the University of Iowa, and through state and local connections.

This letter highlights a few of the many the challenges facing nursing home social services workers and departments during COVID-19. We share them as the challenges, sacrifices, and important work of this professional group was largely unnoticed by the media and may not be widely known even within the social work field. Our group's activities also highlight the ways that researchers can support our practice colleagues at this difficult time, amplify their every-day efforts, and contribute to healing during this pandemic.

Nancy Kusmaul

ⓘ http://orcid.org/0000-0003-2278-8495

Mercedes Bern-Klug

Jennifer Heston-Mullins

Amy R. Roberts

Colleen Galambos

References

Bern-Klug, M., Connolly, R., Downes, D., Galambos, C., Kusmaul, N., Kane, R., Hector, P., & Beaulieu, E. (2016). Responding to the 2015 CMS proposed rule changes for LTC facilities: A call to redouble efforts to prepare students and practitioners for nursing homes. *Journal of Gerontological Social Work, 59*(2), 98–127. https://doi.org/10.1080/01634372.2016.1157116

University of Iowa School of Social Work. (n.d.). *The national nursing home social work network.* https://clas.uiowa.edu/socialwork/nursing-home/national-nursing-home-social-work-network

Working with Older Caregivers of Persons with Mental Illness during COVID-19: Decreasing Burden, Creating Plans for Future Care, and Utilizing Strengths

Dear Editor,

It is estimated that there are 8.4 million caregivers of adults with mental illness in the U.S., with approximately one-half being parents of care recipients (National Alliance for Caregiving, 2015, 2016). Mental illness occurs across the life course and many mental disorders resulting in the need for caregiving are often experienced chronically. As a result, the average caregiver for persons with mental illness is in their mid-50s and approximately one-third – or 2.8 million caregivers – are 60 years of age or older (Lerner et al., 2018; National Alliance for Caregiving, 2016). Below, we argue that during the COVID-19 pandemic, older caregivers of persons with mental illness are particularly likely to experience three challenges and we make recommendations for how social workers can effectively intervene in these areas.

General caregiving burden

While caregiving for persons with mental illness can be a source of growth for caregivers and provide them with rewards and gratifications (Shiraishi & Reilly, 2019), caregiving can also lead to substantial objective and subjective burden (Awad & Voruganti, 2008; Labrum, 2018a). Subjective burden – including psychological distress – is generally associated with managing problematic behaviors of persons with mental illness, level of caregiving provided, and the presence of additional life stressors, such as age-related caregiver health problems (Awad & Voruganti, 2008; Baronet, 1999; Lerner et al., 2018). Shelter at home requirements, related to the COVID-19 pandemic, mean caregivers and care recipients are spending more time together, thus placing pressure on caregivers to provide additional care and supervision, surely exacerbating caregiving burden. Clinician-led family psychoeducation, which entails providing therapeutic support and education about mental illness and caregiving, has been found to have a range of positive effects (Lucksted et al., 2012), including when delivered via the internet (Rotondi et al., 2010). Peer-led family psychoeducation – such as the Family-to-Family program offered through the National Alliance on Mental Illness (NAMI) – has also been found to positively impact caregivers (Dixon et al., 2011). During the COVID-19 pandemic, it is particularly important that social workers connect older caregivers of persons with mental illness to evidence-based family psychoeducational interventions, offered either at community mental health organizations or peer-led support organizations (such as NAMI or Mental Health America, both of which are currently expanding their internet-delivered services).

Future care of persons with mental illness

A significant source of psychological distress for older caregivers is not having plans in place for the care of their loved one after they are no longer able to provide care (Rose et al., 2006). Caregivers of persons with mental illness are less likely to have plans for future care than other caregivers (National Alliance for Caregiving, 2020), and as much as 60% of older caregivers of persons with mental illness may not have such plans (Labrum, 2018b). As older caregivers of persons with mental illness (many of whom may have underlying medical conditions as well as being older) are at an increased risk of severe illness should they contract COVID-19 (Centers for Disease Control and Prevention, 2020), their fears of being unable to provide future care may be more pronounced during the pandemic, and those without plans are likely experiencing considerable distress. It is critical that social workers recognize this and assist older caregivers and care recipients in creating plans for future care. Many caregivers are over-whelmed with navigating care provider systems and social workers should assist persons with mental illness in accessing a range of formal services (e.g., supportive housing, intensive case management, respite care, socialization programs, and professionally provided money management) and, possibly, creating psychiatric advanced directives. Social workers should also help caregivers and persons with mental illness create plans for future care provided by informal support members. Older caregivers often hope that siblings will adopt a caregiving role (Smith et al., 2000), with siblings being more likely to do so if they perceive their sibling with mental illness has reciprocated support (Horwitz, 1994). As most persons with mental illness actively make contributions to family members (Labrum, 2020), it is advisable that social workers assist family members in identifying the contributions they have received from persons with mental illness.

Unmet needs for support among older caregivers

Due to the stigma of mental illness and caregivers having inadequate time to socialize, caregivers of persons with mental illness often experience losses in social relationships and social isolation (Gater et al., 2014; Hayes et al., 2015; Vasileiou et al., 2017). Consequently, they are more likely to have unmet needs for emotional and instrumental support, which are likely exacerbated during the COVID-19 pandemic. Not only is the need for emotional support among older caregivers likely increased due to pandemic-related stressors, restrictions to in-person contact with informal and formal supports may serve as barriers to older caregivers meeting their needs for emotional and instrumental support. While persons with mental illness are more likely to receive than provide support (Haselden et al., 2018; Labrum, 2020), the two are not mutually exclusive (Horwitz et al., 1996; Labrum, 2020), and evidence suggests that more than half of older caregivers receive support with activities of daily living (e.g. completing household chores and grocery shopping) by care recipients with mental illness (Greenberg, 1995); the proportion receiving emotional support and valued companionship is likely considerably greater (Horwitz, 1994; Schwartz & Gidron, 2002). Social workers should recognize that care recipients with mental illness can be an important source of emotional and instrumental support for older caregivers and seek to include both caregivers and persons with mental illness in services. Older caregivers and persons with mental illness should be assisted in identifying how persons with mental illness can provide support and in resolving potential barriers to delivering such support. Care recipients with mental illness often reside with caregivers (National Alliance for Caregiving, 2016), and it is important to remember that they may be particularly apt for providing forms of support to older caregivers that require physical proximity (e.g. assistance with household chores and in-person companionship).

Conclusion

Older caregivers of persons with mental illness are a vulnerable population at risk of experiencing considerable challenges during the COVID-19 pandemic. Social workers are well positioned to work with caregivers and persons with mental illness to ameliorate caregiver burden, create plans for the future care of persons with mental illness, and assist persons with mental illness in providing emotional and instrumental support to older caregivers.

Travis Labrum

Christina Newhill

Tyler Smathers

References

Awad, A. G., & Voruganti, L. N. (2008). The burden of schizophrenia on caregivers. *Pharmacoeconomics*, *26*(2), 149–162. https://doi.org/10.2165/00019053-200826020-00005

Baronet, A. M. (1999). Factors associated with caregiver burden in mental illness A critical review of the research literature. *Clinical Psychology Review*, *19*(7), 819–841. https://doi.org/10.1016/S0272-7358(98)00076-2

Centers for Disease Control and Prevention. (2020). *Groups at higher risk for severe illness.* https://www.cdc.gov/coronavirus/2019-ncov/need-extra-precautions/groups-at-higher-risk.html

Dixon, L. B., Lucksted, A., Medoff, D. R., Burland, J., Stewart, B., Lehman, A. F., Fang, L. J., Sturm, V., Brown, C., & Murray-Swank, A. (2011). Outcomes of a randomized study of a peer-taught family-to-family education program for mental illness. *Psychiatric Services*, *62*(6), 591–597. https://doi.org/10.1176/ps.62.6.pss6206_0591

Gater, A., Rofail, D., Tolley, C., Marshall, C., Abetz-Webb, L., Zarit, S. H., & Berardo, C. G. (2014). Sometimes it's difficult to have a normal life: results from a qualitative study exploring caregiver burden in schizophrenia. *Schizophrenia Research and Treatment*, 368215. https://doi.org/10.1155/2014/368215

Greenberg, J. S. (1995). The other side of caring: Adult children with mental illness as supports to their mothers in later life. *Social Work*, *40*(3), 414–423. https://doi.org/10.1093/sw/40.3.414

Haselden, M., Dixon, L. B., Overley, A., Cohen, A. N., Glynn, S. M., Drapalski, A., Piscitelli, S., & Thorning, H. (2018). Giving back to families: Evidence and predictors of persons with serious mental illness contributing help and support to families. *Community Mental Health Journal*, *54*(4), 383–394. https://doi.org/10.1007/s10597-017-0172-1

Hayes, L., Hawthorne, G., Farhall, J., O'Hanlon, B., & Harvey, C. (2015). Quality of life and social isolation among caregivers of adults with schizophrenia: Policy and outcomes. *Community Mental Health Journal*, *51*(5), 591–597. https://doi.org/10.1007/s10597-015-9848-6

Horwitz, A. V. (1994). Predictors of adult sibling social support for the seriously mentally ill: An exploratory study. *Journal of Family Issues*, *15*, 272–289. https://doi.org/10.1177/0192513X94015002007

Horwitz, A. V., Reinhard, S. C., & Howell-White, S. (1996). Caregiving as reciprocal exchange in families with seriously mentally ill members. *Journal of Health and Social Behavior*, *37*(2), 149–162. https://doi.org/10.2307/2137270

Labrum, T. (2018a). Caregiving for relatives with psychiatric disorders vs. co-occurring psychiatric and substance use disorders. *Psychiatric Quarterly*, *89*(3), 631–644. https://doi.org/10.1007/s11126-017-9557-0

Labrum, T. (2018b). Plans held by older caregivers for the future care of relatives with serious mental illness. *Innovation in Aging*, *2*(suppl_1), 294. https://doi.org/10.1093/geroni/igy023.1084

Labrum, T. (2020). Persons with serious mental illness help relatives: Rates and correlates of assistance. *Journal of Mental Health*, *29*(3), 328–335. Advanced online publication. https://doi.org/10.1080/09638237.2020.1739246

Lerner, D., Chang, H., Rogers, W. H., Benson, C., Lyson, M. C., & Dixon, L. B. (2018). Psychological distress among caregivers of individuals with a diagnosis of schizophrenia or schizoaffective disorder. *Psychiatric Services*, *69*(2), 169–178. https://doi.org/10.1176/appi.ps.201600422

Lucksted, A., McFarlane, W., Downing, D., & Dixon, L. (2012). Recent developments in family psychoeducation as an evidence-based practice. *Journal of Marital and Family Therapy, 38* (1), 101–121. https://doi.org/10.1111/j.1752-0606.2011.00256.x

National Alliance for Caregiving. (2015). *Caregiving in the U.S. 2015.* https://www. caregiving.org/wp-content/uploads/2015/05/2015_CaregivingintheUS_Final-Report-June-4_WEB.pdf

National Alliance for Caregiving. (2016). *On pins and needles: Caregivers of adults with mental illness.* https://www.caregiving.org/wp-content/uploads/2020/05/NAC_Mental_Illness_Study_2016_FINAL_WEB.pdf

National Alliance for Caregiving. (2020). *Caregiving in the U.S. 2020.* https://www.caregiving. org/wp-content/uploads/2020/05/Full-Report-Caregiving-in-the-United-States-2020.pdf

Rose, L. E., Mallinson, R. K., & Gerson, L. D. (2006). Mastery, burden, and areas of concern among family caregivers of mentally ill persons. *Archives of Psychiatric Nursing, 20*(1), 41–51. https://doi.org/10.1016/j.apnu.2005.08.009

Rotondi, A. J., Anderson, C. M., Haas, G. L., Eack, S. M., Spring, M. B., Ganguli, R., Newhill, C. E., & Rosenstock, J. (2010). Web-based psychoeducational intervention for persons with schizophrenia and their supporters: One-year outcomes. *Psychiatric Services, 61*(11), 1099–1105. https://doi.org/10.1176/ps.2010.61.11.1099

Schwartz, C., & Gidron, R. (2002). Parents of mentally ill adult children living at home: Rewards of caregiving. *Health & Social Work, 27*(2), 145–154. https://doi.org/10.1093/hsw/27.2.145

Shiraishi, N., & Reilly, J. (2019). Positive and negative impacts of schizophrenia on family caregivers: A systematic review and qualitative meta-summary. *Social Psychiatry and Psychiatric Epidemiology, 54*(3), 277–290. https://doi.org/10.1007/s00127-018-1617-8

Smith, G. C., Hatfield, A. B., & Miller, D. C. (2000). Planning by older mothers for the future care of offspring with serious mental illness. *Psychiatric Services, 51*(9), 1162–1166. https://doi.org/10.1176/appi.ps.51.9.1162

Vasileiou, K., Barnett, J., Barreto, M., Vines, J., Atkinson, M., Lawson, S., & Wilson, M. (2017). Experiences of loneliness associated with being an informal caregiver: A qualitative investigation. *Frontiers in Psychology, 8.* https://doi.org/10.3389/fpsyg.2017.00585

Service Needs of Older Adults with Serious Mental Illness

Dear Editor,

As the global population ages, the mental health workforce must adapt to serve the growing number of older adults with serious mental illnesses (OASMI) such as schizophrenia, bipolar, and major depressive disorders. OASMI may have complex needs related to physical, psychological, and social well-being. Social workers with skills in diagnosis, care coordination, delivery of evidence-based practices, and knowledge of community resources can play an important role in meeting these needs (Olfson, 2016). The COVID-19 pandemic makes the need to better serve this population even more urgent, as OASMI have higher rates of chronic health conditions and tobacco use and more limited support networks, which increase susceptibility to complications associated with COVID-19 (Druss, 2020). This letter aims to inform social workers of the health and psychosocial needs of OASMI and interventions to support well-being.

Physical, social, and emotional needs interact to amplify distress and increase risk of mortality among adults 50 and older with SMI. Persons with SMI have high rates of trauma exposure and post-traumatic stress (Lewis et al., 2018). Exposure to chronic stressors may increase allostatic load – the cumulative effect of stress resulting in biological dysregulation – which may accelerate biological aging and contribute to physical health conditions (Juster et al., 2010). Disparities in health-care, lifestyle choices, and effects of psychotropic medications complicate self-management of health conditions like diabetes and cardiovascular disease. Loneliness is important to consider during this time of social distancing; through its positive association with depressive symptoms, it may indirectly contribute to thoughts of self-harm among OASMI Dell, et al., (2019, 2020). Social skill deficits can contribute to loneliness, and complicate communication with healthcare providers, increasing the risk of health problems (Segrin, 2017). Healthcare providers may stigmatize old age and mental illness (Benjenk et al., 2019), which, if internalized, can contribute to poorer social functioning (Muñoz et al., 2011).

In addition to providing psychoeducation and normalizing common emotional reactions like fear or anxiety in response to the pandemic, social workers may promote well-being through psychosocial skills training, illness-self management, and collaborative care interventions (Bartels et al., 2018). Integrated community care models and lifestyle interventions have been associated with reduced excess mortality among persons with SMI (Baxter et al., 2016). Well-being may also be enhanced through cognitive stimulation and remediation, positive psychology and mindfulness approaches, and social engagement (Harmell et al., 2014). A recent review identified 14 multidimensional wellness interventions for OASMI primarily addressing physical, social, emotional, and environmental domains of wellness, but found little evidence that these have been widely adopted in inpatient, outpatient, or geriatric medical settings (Zechner et al., 2019).

The United States' Substance Abuse and Mental Health Services Administration (2019) identified several workforce-related barriers to serving OASMI, which increase OASMI's vulnerability to poorer outcomes: a shortage of mental health providers with geriatric expertise, lack of incentives to enter the field, limited training opportunities, and lack of support for caregivers and direct care workers. Mental health professionals may need support in acquiring the knowledge and skill to operate within collaborative, integrated primary and behavioral healthcare settings. During the pandemic, mobile health technologies may enhance psychiatric rehabilitation services that have been disrupted, as agencies transition to provide more telehealth services (Bartels et al., 2018).

The effects of the pandemic amplify the vulnerabilities OASMI already experience. Providers may leverage mobile and telehealth technologies to ensure continuity in care and promote psychosocial functioning. Social workers serving OASMI may consider how to implement integrated care models to address the cumulative effects of trauma and chronic stress contributing to chronic physical and mental health conditions placing clients at greater risk for COVID-19.

Nathaniel A. Dell

(iD) http://orcid.org/0000-0003-3055-6301

Natsuki Sasaki

(iD) http://orcid.org/0000-0001-8813-1432

Madeline Stewart

Allison M. Murphy and Marina Klier

References

Bartels, S. J., DiMilia, P. R., Fortuna, K. L., & Naslund, J. A. (2018). Integrated care for older adults with serious mental illness and medical comorbidity: Evidence-based models and future research directions. *Psychiatric Clinics*, *41*(1), 153–164. https://doi.org/10.1016/j.psc. 2017.10.012

Baxter, A., Harris, M., Khatib, Y., Brugha, T., Bien, H., & Bhui, K. (2016). Reducing excess mortality due to chronic disease in people with severe mental illness: Meta-review of health interventions. *British Journal Of Psychiatry*, *208*(4), 322–329. https://doi.org/10.1192/bjp.bp. 115.163170

Benjenk, I., Buchongo, P., Amaize, A., Martinez, G. S., & Chen, J. (2019). Overcoming the dual stigma of mental illness and aging: Preparing new nurses to care for the mental health needs of older adults. *The American Journal of Geriatric Psychiatry, 27*(7), 664–674. https://doi.org/10.1016/j.jagp.2018.12.028

Dell, N. A., Huang, J., Buttafuoco, K., Vidovic, K., Murphy, A., & Farrar, L. (2020). Direct and indirect associations between loneliness and thoughts of self-harm among persons with serious mental illness.

Dell, N. A, Pelham, M, & Murphy, A. M. (2019). Loneliness and depressive symptoms in middle aged and older adults experiencing serious mental illness. *Psychiatric Rehabilitation Journal, 42*(2), 113-120. doi: 10.1037/prj0000347

Druss, B. G. (2020). Addressing the COVID-19 pandemic in populations with serious mental illness. *JAMA Psychiatry (Chicago, Ill.).* Published online April 03, 2020. https://doi.org/10.1001/jamapsychiatry.2020.0894

Harmell, A. L., Jeste, D., & Depp, C. (2014). Strategies for successful aging: A research update. *Current Psychiatry Reports, 16*(10), 476. https://doi.org/10.1007/s11920-014-0476-6

Juster, R. P., McEwen, B. S., & Lupien, S. J. (2010). Allostatic load biomarkers of chronic stress and impact on health and cognition. *Neuroscience and Biobehavioral Reviews, 35*(1), 2–16. https://doi.org/10.1016/j.neubiorev.2009.10.002

Lewis, C., Raisanen, L., Bisson, J. I., Jones, I., & Zammit, S. (2018). Trauma exposure and undetected posttraumatic stress disorder among adults with a mental disorder. *Depression and Anxiety, 35*(2), 178–184. https://doi.org/10.1002/da.22707

Muñoz, M., Sanz, M., Pérez-Santos, E., & de Los Ángeles Quiroga, M. (2011). Proposal of a socio–cognitive–behavioral structural equation model of internalized stigma in people with severe and persistent mental illness. *Psychiatry Research, 186*(2–3), 402–408. https://doi.org/10.1016/j.psychres.2010.06.019

Olfson, M. (2016). Building the mental health workforce capacity needed to treat adults with serious mental illnesses. *Health Affairs, 35*(6), 983–990. https://doi.org/10.1377/hlthaff.2015.1619

Segrin, C. (2019). Indirect effects of social skills on health through stress and loneliness. *Health Communication, 34*(1), 118–124. https://doi.org/10.1080/10410236.2017.1384434

Substance Abuse and Mental Health Services Administration. (2019). *Older adults living with serious mental illness: The state of the behavioral health workforce.* Author. Retrieved from: https://store.samhsa.gov/product/Older-Adults-Living-with-Serious-Mental-Illness-The-State-of-the-Behavioral-Health-Workforce/PEP19-OLDERADULTS-SMI

Zechner, M., Pratt, C., Barrett, N., Dreker, M., & Santos, S. (2019). Multi-dimensional wellness interventions for older adults with serious mental illness: A systematic literature review. *Psychiatric Rehabilitation Journal, 42*(4), 382–393. https://doi.org/10.1037/prj0000342

The Implications of COVID-19 for the Mental Health Care of Older Adults: Insights from Emergency Department Social Workers

Dear Editor,

The increased number of older adults with mental health needs, combined with a shortage of geriatric mental health professionals, is a growing crisis in American health care. The ongoing COVID-19 pandemic and measures to contain and mitigate its spread will likely exacerbate this crisis. In this letter, we discuss the possible ways in which the pandemic may disrupt geriatric mental health, incorporating the experience of two frontline social workers in emergency departments (EDs), including one in psychiatric emergency services (PES) program within an ED. EDs are a major entry point into the mental health care system and an important location for referrals to community services. Social workers are a crucial part of the interdisciplinary medical team in the ED that provides critical services such as assessment, treatment, care coordination, and referrals to patients with complex health and social care needs.

An impact of the pandemic already felt by frontline social workers is the disruptions to mental health care access and delivery. Changes in staffing, physical capacity, and clinical workflows in various health care settings have occurred due to hospital infection-control measures, diversion of resources toward COVID-19 care, and financial pressures. These changes may cause delays across different points in the care continuum. We have seen longer wait times for psychiatric patients to get evaluated and admitted as they wait for COVID-19 test results, which could take as long as 12 hours. Patients may experience additional delays in receiving inpatient care due to shortages of psychiatric beds, an existing problem that is worsened by the pandemic. In one of our practice settings, the number of psychiatric beds has been halved due to hospital social distancing measures, which has sometimes resulted in transfers to other hospitals as far as 2 hours away. Further complicating discharge planning, many skilled nursing facilities are hesitant to take patients directly from EDs and may require one or more negative COVID-19 tests before acceptance. These bottlenecks in care transitions not only pose challenges to social workers but may also lead to poor patient outcomes, medical errors, readmissions, and increased health care costs (Naylor & Keating, 2008). These negative impacts are likely to be pronounced for older adults with complex medical and mental health needs. These inefficiencies may also impact the wellbeing of family caregivers. We have seen increased levels of anxiety, stress, and feelings of guilt from family members as they conduct caregiving remotely. Due to visitor restrictions, families may be unable to provide information that could meaningfully inform treatment and discharge planning.

The pandemic is likely to increase the number of older adults with mental health needs, including those new to the mental health care system and those experiencing an exacerbation in their existing psychiatric conditions. Although relevant data are sparse, a recent American Psychiatric Association poll found high levels of COVID-19-related anxiety, with over one-third of American adults believing that coronavirus is having a serious impact on their mental health (Canady, 2020). A coauthor's PES unit has seen an increase in calls to their crisis phone services and walk-ins for anxiety-related concerns among older adults. Patients with chronic and severe mental illness may experience acute psychotic episodes related to COVID-19 (Fischer et al., 2020).

Besides COVID-19-related anxiety and paranoia, control measures such as social distancing, business closures, and stay-at-home orders may lead to social isolation and loneliness, which can increase the risk of depression and anxiety (Santini et al., 2020). These mental health consequences may be pronounced for older adults who live alone, especially those who lack technology that can help in maintaining social connections. Older adults residing in multigenerational households may experience increased conflicts at home, which may worsen mental health and wellbeing. Those who are in abusive relationships may experience an exacerbation of this abuse (Campbell, 2020). Cases of complicated grief may also increase, as the number of deaths climbs and disruptions to familiar ways of grieving continue. Related to pandemic control is the cancellation of most elective surgeries, which can have adverse mental health consequences. We have seen in our clinics an increase in feelings of hopelessness among patients with canceled surgeries, especially when they had waited months for a surgery date and for procedures to relieve painful conditions and improve quality of life. Some older adults may avoid seeking care altogether, even when medically urgent and necessary (Moroni et al., 2020). Additionally, the stock market volatility and the high unemployment rate due to the pandemic may adversely affect the financial wellbeing of older adults, particularly for those who are nearing retirement. This socioeconomic decline can lead to a variety of mental health problems such as depression, anxiety, substance use, and suicide.

The COVID-19 pandemic likely will have profound impacts on the mental health of older adults by increasing their demand for services while disrupting the supply of high-quality and timely care. Understanding the extent and duration of the mental health impacts and identification of best practices will require carefully planned observational studies and experimentations. In the meantime, social workers across care settings can contribute to knowledge building by documenting the measures taken to prevent and address the mental health needs of older adults and families in their practices and, as permitted, collect data for evaluation.

Xiaoling Xiang

http://orcid.org/0000-0002-4926-4707

Yawen Ning

Jay Kayser

References

Campbell, A. M. (2020). An increasing risk of family violence during the Covid-19 pandemic: Strengthening community collaborations to save lives. *Forensic Science International: Reports.* https://doi.org/10.1016/j.fsir.2020.100089

Canady, V. A. (2020). APA poll finds nearly half anxious about getting COVID-19. *Mental Health Weekly.* https://doi.org/10.1002/mhw.32295

Fischer, M., Coogan, A. N., Faltraco, F., & Thome, J. (2020). COVID-19 paranoia in a patient suffering from schizophrenic psychosis – A case report. *Psychiatry Research, 288*, 113001. https://doi.org/10.1016/j.psychres.2020.113001

Moroni, F., Gramegna, M., Ajello, S., Beneduce, A., Baldetti, L., Vilca, L. M., Cappelletti, A., Scandroglio, A. M., & Azzalini, L. (2020). Collateral damage: Medical care avoidance behavior among patients with acute coronary syndrome during the COVID-19 pandemic. *JACC: Case Reports.* https://doi.org/10.1016/j.jaccas.2020.04.010

Naylor, M., & Keating, S. A. (2008). Transitional care: Moving patients from one care setting to another. *The American Journal of Nursing.* https://doi.org/10.1097/01.NAJ.0000336420.34946.3a

Santini, Z. I., Jose, P. E., York Cornwell, E., Koyanagi, A., Nielsen, L., Hinrichsen, C., Meilstrup, C., Madsen, K. R., & Koushede, V. (2020). Social disconnectedness, perceived isolation, and symptoms of depression and anxiety among older Americans (NSHAP): A longitudinal mediation analysis. *The Lancet Public Health, 5*(1), e62–e70. https://doi.org/10.1016/S2468-2667(19)30230-0

Psychosocial Impact of COVID-19 on Older Adults: A Cultural Geriatric Mental Health-Care Perspectived

Dear Editor,

The COVID-19 pandemic has claimed 335 thousand lives with 5.15 million confirmed cases across 213 countries and territories to date. The fatality rate of COVID-19 by age is higher in sexagenarians (14.8%), septuagenarians (8.0%), and octogenarians (3.6%) as of the date of this paper is written. China, with the largest aging population, has the highest number of associated deaths in older adults. At present, Pakistan has 11.3 million people (15.8%) of the world population. By 2050, it is estimated that about fifth of the Pakistan population will be aged 65 years and older (Haleem et al., 2020). However, there is currently very little known about the broader impact of COVID-19 on global mental health, in general, and geriatric mental health, in particular. Mental health concerns are common in older adults with the prevalent depressive symptoms. The rapid transmission of COVID-19 in this pandemic outbreak, higher mortality rates, self-isolation, social-distancing, and quarantine could all exacerbate the risk of mental health difficulties (Mukhtar, 2020a). Mental health issues (new or existing) could worsen and further impair the cognitive and emotional functioning of persons of all ages. The impact of mental health difficulties on older adults varies around the world and the factors impacting geriatric mental health could differ from low-middle income countries (LMICs) to developed countries. Pakistan being a collectivistic culture depends highly on an extended joint filial and fraternal family system. The predominant role of older adults, especially grand-relatives, includes group dining, seeking social-cohesion, and family support through multiple events led by older members of the family. Additionally, a family's social and economic dependence on older adults and the decision-making of household through older adults is one of the main tenants in Pakistan's cultural system.

Unlike the young segment of the population which is efficiently equipped with modern technologies and internet services – awareness of smartphones and technology literacy disparity is low among most older adults. The use of social media can act as a tool to prevent loneliness, boredom, and tediousness in young group but for the older age group the need of social support, liveliness, and daily functioning remain unmet. Online technologies and digital sources are now harnessed to provide virtual-digital social support networks and a perceived sense of belonging (Mukhtar, 2020b). The mass quarantine and transport restraints in Pakistan have inevitably constricted the activities of older adults: regular walk-and-talk in the park, acquaintance meetings, voluntary service and social care, congregational gatherings, contact with plants and animals, and obtaining prescribed nutrition, medication, and treatment. Thus, these are further aggravating challenges in the wake of COVID-19 for the positive mental health of older adults in the community. Globally, insufficient and inadequate attention has been paid to the mental health of older age groups in terms of quality and timely psychological crisis intervention.

Self-isolation, social-distancing, social disconnectedness, and loneliness were found to be linked to depression and anxiety in a similar recent study (Rana et al., 2020). Self-perceived social disconnectedness and perceived isolation have predicted higher depressive and anxiety symptoms (Mukhtar, 2020a). Brief evidence-based psychological preventive public health interventions could be established and implemented within the residential environment, health-care facilities, nursing centers, religious and cultural organizations, and social and community centers for older adults (Mukhtar, 2020b). Action-based psychological preventive public health strategies could cultivate social connection and promote healthy relationships with one's own-self and others. Cognitive skills and social support networks could help older adults to foster meaningful connection and sense of belongingness during this isolation period. Cognitive, behavioral, social, positive, and brief therapies delivered online or in-person could enhance mental wellbeing (Mukhtar, 2020d). These may further improve social affiliation and support while simultaneously diminishing perceived loneliness.

Social isolation and social disconnection – their documented bidirectional and complex relationship between mental health issues and social disconnectedness – poses a serious public health concern among older adults. This is due to psychosocial issues and physiological health problems such as mental health problems, diabetes, cardiovascular, autoimmune, neurocognitive, neurobiological, and other at-risk health problems (Mukhtar, 2020c; Mukhtar & Mukhtar, 2020). States and global health organizations should establish mental health policies for older people who are socially isolated at home or quarantined at health-care facilities (hospital, clinic, isolation unit, daycare, community center, and place of worship) for not only prescribed diet and medications but their mental health care as well (Mukhtar & Rana, 2020). They should be communicated with about the meaning of coronavirus-related social preventive measures to mitigate their physical and mental health consequences. While adherence to social isolation strategies could weaken with time, well-timed geriatric social service intervention could efficiently prevent the morbidity related to geriatric mental health care.

Sonia Mukhtar

iD http://orcid.org/0000-0003-4480-648X

Acknowledgments

My gratitude goes to my "younger from heart" friends for sharing information about their current situations.

Declaration of competing interest

The authors declare no conflict of interest.

References

Haleem, A., Javaid, M., & Vaishya, R. (2020). Effects of COVID-19 pandemic in daily life. *CMRP (10)* 2. https://doi.org/10.1016/j.cmrp.2020.03.011

Mukhtar, S. (2020a). Mental health and emotional impact of COVID-19: Applying health belief model for medical staff to general public of Pakistan. *Brain, Behavior, and Immunity*, S0889-1591(20)30463-3. https://doi.org/10.1016/j.bbi.2020.04.012

Mukhtar, S. (2020b). Mental health and psychosocial aspects of coronavirus outbreak in Pakistan: Psychological intervention for public mental health crisis. *Asian Journal of Psychiatry*, *51*, 102069. https://doi.org/10.1016/j.ajp.2020.102069

Mukhtar, S. (2020c). Pakistanis' mental health during the COVID-19. *Asian Journal of Psychiatry*, *51*, 102127. https://doi.org/10.1016/j.ajp.2020.102127

Mukhtar, S. (2020d). Psychological health during the coronavirus disease 2019 pandemic outbreak. *International Journal of Social Psychiatry*, 002076402092583. https://doi.org/10.1177/0020764020925835

Mukhtar, S., & Mukhtar, S. (2020). Letter to the editor: Mental health and psychological distress in people with diabetes during COVID-19. *Metabolism*, *108*, 154248. https://doi.org/10.1016/j.metabol.2020.154248

Mukhtar, S., & Rana, W. (2020). COVID-19 and individuals with mental illness in psychiatric facilities. *Psychiatry Research*, *289*, 113075. https://doi.org/10.1016/j.psychres.2020.113075

Rana, W., Mukhtar, S., & Mukhtar, S. (2020). Mental health of medical workers in Pakistan during the pandemic COVID-19 outbreak. *Asian Journal of Psychiatry*, *51*, 102080. https://doi.org/10.1016/j.ajp.2020.102080

Part V

Social Isolation and the Digital Experience in COVID-19

Practical Implications of Physical Distancing, Social Isolation, and Reduced Physicality for Older Adults in Response to COVID-19

Dear Editor,

Images and stories emerging from the novel coronavirus (COVID-19) pandemic illustrate the importance of human relationships in societies across the globe. Scenes such as family members holding vigil outside nursing home windows where their loved ones are quarantined, funerals and burials being held without mourners present, and people isolated from their families and communities for extended time periods demonstrate the unprecedented nature of the social impacts of responding to an international health crisis. The pandemic has affected the lives of older adults and their families across the world and how social workers can help them, with examples such as increased reliance on kinship care networks as alternative care in Ghana (Cudjoe & Abdullah, 2020) and mounting concerns about vulnerable older adults with limited resources during social isolation in India (Nagarkar, 2020). Given the immense reach and scale of the COVID-19 pandemic, social workers must emphasize and advocate for the universal importance of social connections and the dire consequences of social isolation, particularly for older adults.

The novel coronavirus brought with it a concept novel to most – "social distancing." At an astonishing pace, social distancing became a ubiquitous catchphrase used to refer to a key strategy to reduce potential exposure to the virus. The actual intention of social distancing is to reduce *physical* contact between people to limit viral transmission. While the misnomered term social distancing is now firmly fixed into mainstream vernacular, social workers should advocate for the use the more accurate language of "physical distancing."

Despite the public health benefit of physical distancing in reducing community spread, the implemented measures have produced a perfect storm of social disruptions with tremendous implications for the health and well-being of older adults. The obvious implication involves the potential for increased social isolation which is associated with both poorer physical and mental health outcomes and loneliness (Brown & Munson, 2020). Separation from family, friends, and larger communities is often accompanied by reduced ability to engage in meaningful activities and relationships that lead to one's sense of self-worth (Drageset et al., 2015). Furthermore, with older adults with preexisting medical conditions being considered an at-risk population, there is an increased need to self-isolate due to heightened health concerns. These physical and social separations from loved ones during a time of hardship for many may lead to complicated grief and loss experiences, including the experience of individual and collective trauma reactions.

The consequences of physical distancing will affect older adults across all environments from independent community living to those living in long-term care facilities. Independent older adults may experience disruptions in their daily active routines that require major adjustments. Community-dwelling older adults who need some assistance may experience a loss of instrumental social support including direct physical assistance with food procurement, access to medications, assistance with daily household tasks, and assistance with access to informal and formal health care services (which also may be disrupted). Reduced social interaction in long-term care facilities may involve suspension of visitation, shared meals, and group activities, reduced connection to religious communities, and limited opportunities for physical activity. Much of the effects of physical distancing are related to the idea that social relationships involve a great degree of physicality. Sharing physical space and touch is a valuable feature of relationships with family and friends, with connection and love often expressed through eye contact, hand-shakes, hugs, or other forms of physical expression. To offset some of these limitations, social contact with others via telephone or web-based video technologies may help maintain social connections but the quality of these contacts is reduced compared to face-to-face, physical interactions and some older adults may not have access to such technologies (Seifert, 2020).

For sure, there will be additional unforeseen consequences of physical distancing and social isolation as a result of this pandemic. All of the implications listed above may be more intense for marginalized older adults such as those in lower socioeconomic status, rural, minority, and LGBTQ populations, who were already experiencing the effects of social isolation and health disparities. Lessons to be learned from this pandemic include the reminders that all human beings are intrinsically linked by social ties and intergenerational connections and the actions of younger generations directly impact the health and well-being of older adult and vulnerable populations. Indeed, the COVID-19 pandemic has sparked a renewed interest in ideas related to social isolation and social support. Social workers are tasked with identifying policy and practice approaches for helping older adults maintain resilient social connections in times of duress and envisioning how communities and greater society can respond to social challenges in future pandemics.

Anthony D. Campbell

References

Brown, S., & Munson, M. R. (2020). Introduction to the special issue on social isolation across the lifespan. *Clinical Social Work Journal, 48*(1), 1–5. https://doi.org/10.1007/s10615-020-00750-3

Cudjoe, E., & Abdullah, A. (2020). Drawing on kinship care support for older people during a pandemic (COVID-19): Practice considerations for social workers in Ghana. *Journal of Gerontological Social Work*, 1–3. https://doi.org/10.1080/01634372.2020.1758271

Drageset, J., Eide, G. E., Dysvik, E., Furnes, B., & Hauge, S. (2015). Loneliness, loss, and social support among cognitively intact older people with cancer, living in nursing homes – A mixed-methods study. *Clinical Interventions in Aging, 10*, 1529-1536. https://doi.org/10.2147/CIA.588404

Nagarkar, A. (2020). Challenges and concerns for older adults in India regarding the COVID-19 pandemic. *Journal of Gerontological Social Work*, 1–3. https://doi.org/10.1080/01634372.2020.1763534

Seifert, A. (2020). The digital exclusion of older adults during the COVID-19 pandemic. *Journal of Gerontological Social Work*, 1–3. https://doi.org/10.1080/01634372.2020.1764687

COVID-19 and the Digital Divide: Will Social Workers Help Bridge the Gap?

Dear Editor,

The COVID-19 pandemic has impacted almost every facet of life. For social work professionals, the implementation of social distancing policies have altered how we interact with clients. While many areas of practice have embraced remote offerings and telehealth, use of such methods with older adults continues to be a challenge. This letter is a call to action for gerontological social workers to make efforts to close the digital divide. This issue is a matter of social justice to ensure the information and resources from technology can be accessed by all. As a profession, we must make strides to ensure individuals of all ages have access to, and the ability to use, the technological resources available to support health and well-being.

The social distancing requirements necessary to reduce and slow the transmission of COVID-19 can be isolating for people of all ages. Older adults are particularly vulnerable to poorer health outcomes from COVID-19 while also being at heightened risk for loneliness and decreased social engagement. Further, those without Internet access/electronic equipment (i.e., smartphones, computers, tablets, etc.) may be unable to receive primary care and other medical services as many are exclusively being offered remotely. This can exacerbate health disparities among this population. During the spring 2020 shutdown in the United States, 1 in 6 older adults delayed or canceled essential medical treatment due to COVID-19 and only 1 in 5 older adults received medical care by phone or video chat (NORC at the University of Chicago, 2020).

In addition to issues with accessing healthcare, contact with family and social supports is also limited or absent. Those in long term care facilities are unable to have visitors. The potential for poor mental health outcomes is high and we must be proactive in finding alternative support. While in-person interactions are restricted, people across the globe are turning to remote strategies for connection. For older adults, many experience limitations in utilizing electronic communication such as financial challenges to accessing/using technology and lack of knowledge and/or comfort to use technology (Charness, 2016; Czaja et al., 2006). Socioeconomic status also plays a substantial role in older adult Internet access (Gracia & Herrero, 2009). The Pew Research Center reports that only half of Americans 65 and older have home Internet (Pew Research Center, 2017). This percentage falls to less than 30% for older adults aged 80 and older (Pew Research Center).

Given what we know about older adults' use of technology, social workers need to identify creative strategies to continue to engage this population. One such approach is supporting older adults through technology training (Leedahl et al., 2019; Mitzner et al., 2008). Evidence suggests that older adults would be more comfortable with and willing to adopt new technologies if they receive some type of formal training (Mitzner et al., 2008). Social workers should explore various strategies, many of which already exist, to assist individuals in learning and using new telehealth and social engagement technologies.

In addition to training, social workers can engage in advocacy efforts to expand technological access for older adults. The social work profession is dedicated to meeting the needs of all people, especially those who are vulnerable or living in poverty. COVID-19 brings to the forefront that many individuals are not receiving needed care and social services. Existing disadvantage seems to be heightened by current circumstances, with COVID disproportionately impacting racial minorities and those in lower socioeconomic areas. Advocacy efforts should also include efforts to enable equitable access to technology, given the increased role technology now plays in supporting health and wellbeing. While some forms of electronic equipment (i.e., non-smartphones and tablets) are becoming more affordable, they may be inaccessible to older adults with extremely limited or fixed financial resources. Further, the cost to access adequate phone minutes or Internet services continues to be a barrier. Efforts to expand access, provide discounted technology services to seniors, or electronic check-out libraries (e.g., "borrow a tablet") through avenues such as care facilities or senior centers should be explored to increase access to those that may wish to use electronic communication but have limited means.

Social workers must be prepared to respond to COVID-19 and play an active role in making sure basic needs are met and all individuals have access to the resources needed to support their health, including technology. COVID-19 is revealing inequities that we already knew existed, but this crisis has exposed that these disparities can no longer be ignored. Through ingenuity, social workers can ensure that the digital divide does not leave "those without" further behind.

Allison Gibson

ⓘ http://orcid.org/0000-0002-4116-9465

Shoshana H. Bardach

Natalie D. Pope

References

Charness, N. (2016). Constraints on adoption of telehealth to support aging populations. In S. Kwon (Ed.), *Gerontechnology: Research, practice, and principles in the field of technology and aging* (pp. 271–290). Springer Publishing Company.

Czaja, S. J., Charness, N., Fisk, A. D., Hertzog, C., Nair, S. N., Rogers, W. A., & Sharit, J. (2006). Factors predicting the use of technology: Findings from the center for research and education on aging and technology enhancement (CREATE). *Psychology and Aging, 21(2)*, 333–352. https://doi.org/10.1037/0882-7974.21.2.33316768579

Gracia, E., & Herrero, J. (2009). Internet use and self-rated health among older people: A national survey. *Journal of Medical Internet Research, 11*(4), e49. https://doi.org/10.2196/jmir.1311

Leedahl, S. N., Brasher, M., Estus, E., Breck, B. M., Dennis, C. B., & Clark, S. C. (2019). Implementing an interdisciplinary intergenerational program using the Cyber-Seniors ° reverse mentoring model. *Journal of Gerontology & Geriatrics Education, 41*(1), 71–89. https://doi.org/10.1080/02701960.2018.1428574

Mitzner, T. L., Fausset, C. B., Boron, J. B., Adams, A. E., Dijkstra, K., Lee, C. C., & Fisk, A. D. (2008). Older adults' training preferences for learning to use technology. In *Proceedings of the human factors and ergonomics society 52nd annual meeting*, (pp. 2047–2051). Santa Monica, CA: Human Factors and Ergonomics Society.

NORC at the University of Chicago. (2020). *More than half of older adults already experiencing disruptions in care as a result of coronavirus*. University of Chicago. Retrieved from https://www.norc.org/PDFs/JAHF%20TSF/JAHF_TSF_NORC_topline_42720.pdf

Pew Research Center. (2017). *Tech adoption climbs among older adults*. Pew Research Center. Retrieved from https://www.pewresearch.org/internet/2017/05/17/tech-adoption-climbs-among-older-adults/

The Digital Exclusion of Older Adults during the COVID-19 Pandemic

Dear Editor,

During the current worldwide COVID-19 pandemic, older adults are particularly excluded from in-person society on one hand and on the other hand older adults belong to the population group who are often excluded from digital services because they opt to not use new technologies (e.g., smartphones, internet, tablets). This missing digital participation includes also various specifically useful online services and content such as health information, digital social events and social networking or online shopping opportunities. Nonparticipation in the digital world could lead to a doubled feeling of social exclusion in times of physical distancing.

Digital technologies pervade all aspects of our lives. In recent years, we have seen the digitalization of everyday life by high levels of technological innovation. The internet is one of the most important examples of modern digital technology. As internet access has become widespread across the globe, a digital gap between younger and older adults has been observed today in empirical studies (Hunsaker & Hargittai, 2018). Young age groups are currently embracing the internet, whereas adults who have not grown up using these technologies have been observed to use the internet less. For example, one representative study in the US found that only 67% of people 65 years and older were online (Anderson et al., 2019). While the gap in internet use between emerging and advanced economies has narrowed in recent years, there are still regions in the world, especially within developing countries, where significant numbers of older citizens do not use the internet (Pew Research Center, 2018). The situation is not as different in Europe as one might suppose: a representative survey conducted across Switzerland and 16 European Union countries showed that only 49% of people aged 50 years and older used the internet (König et al., 2018). The findings indicated that internet use among older adults was influenced by personal factors, such as age, gender, education, and income. The study showed that people above 80 years spent less time online than people in a slightly lower age group (i.e., 65–79 years). Men and older adults with higher educational and economic status were more likely to use the internet. In addition, individuals' health, prior experience with technology, social salience (internet use among the

---

Special Issue: Letter to the editors: JGSW call for Letters to the Editor: Corona Virus, COVID-19, and social work with older adults

members of one's social network), and contextual factors, such as country-specific wealth and communication technology infrastructure, were predictors of internet usage by older adults.

Access to the internet, or the lack of it, is only one aspect of participation in the digital world. DiMaggio et al. (2004) coined the term digital inequalities to describe this multidimensional digital divide, subdividing it into usage, skills, social support, and self-perception. Usage refers to the variety of different purposes one might have for accessing online content, while skills refers to individuals' internet-specific knowledge. Social support refers to the intensity of support obtained from offline and online networks. Self-perception refers to an individual's personality and his or her attitudes toward internet use. Digital inequality thus refers not only to being "in" or "out" in terms of access to digital technologies but also to participating either actively or passively in the digital society.

Despite the positive outcomes of social participation of people worldwide in the digital world during the COVID-19 pandemic, older adults are at risk of feeling excluded from it. From a sociological perspective, social exclusion is "a multidimensional, relational process of progressive social disengagement, one having interrelated negative consequences for quality of life and well-being of the individual as well as for the quality of society in terms of social cohesion" (Böhnke & Silver, 2014). In the case of internet participation, exclusion means exclusion from a society that is dominated by the internet and digital technologies in many areas of everyday life. The exclusion from participation in these digital areas of everyday life in some cases leads to a subjective feeling of social exclusion (Seifert et al., 2018).

A focus only on digital events as a means of social participation during the COVID-19 pandemic has the potential to perpetuate ageism – that is, older non-users of technology are viewed as outsiders, additional to the already prevailing view of older adults as rendered frail and physically isolated by the COVID-19 pandemic. If inclusion in society nowadays means active participation in the digital world, then older adults who are not online or not active on the internet are at risk of social exclusion. As an increasing number of service providers have to change from personal to virtual information and service provision on an online-only basis, older citizens who are offline could become increasingly disadvantaged as the internet's societal pervasiveness progresses. Society must therefore work together to minimize the risk of social exclusion in relation to digital content on the internet, especially regarding important health information or initiatives for social participation in times of physical distancing. This means that everyone can help to avoid this double exclusion of older adults by, firstly, being sensitive about the digital divide and providing social interaction via "old" technologies such as telephone or letters and, secondly, being creative in bridging the digital divide by, for example, buying a smartphone for their older parents with pre-installed vide-chat apps and sending it to the parents with a point-by-point introduction via telephone. Today being "creative" is not only about being creative on the web with home-office videos but also in connecting older adults with society in offline ways. Little steps, such as ringing parents or older neighbors by telephone or dropping postcards into their letterbox asking them to tick a box concerning the kind of help they most need or asking them if they want help with the purchasing of food, can achieve this. Let's not socially isolate older adults in times of physical distancing; the digital way is one way to connect, but not the way for everyone – we must keep this in mind.

Alexander Seifert

http://orcid.org/0000-0003-3124-4588

References

Anderson, M., Perrin, A., Jiang, J., & Kumar, M. (2019). *10% of Americans don't use the internet. Who are they?* Retrieved November 19, 2019, from Pew Research Center website. https://www.pewresearch.org/fact-tank/2019/04/22/some-americans-dont-use-the-internet-who-are-they/

Böhnke, P., & Silver, H. (2014). Social exclusion. In A. C. Michalos, (Ed..), *Encyclopedia of quality of life and well-being research* (pp. 6064–6069). Dordrecht: Springer Netherlands. https://doi.org/10.1007/978-94-007-0753-5_2757

DiMaggio, P., Hargittai, E., Celeste, C., & Shafer, S. (2004). Digital inequality: From unequal access to differentiated use. In K. M. Neckermann (Ed.), *Social inequality* (pp. 335–400). Russel Sage Foundation.

Hunsaker, A., & Hargittai, E. (2018). A review of Internet use among older adults. *New Media & Society*, 20(10), 3937–3954. https://doi.org/10.1177/1461444818787348

König, R., Seifert, A., & Doh, M. (2018). Internet use among older Europeans: An analysis based on SHARE data. *Universal Access in the Information Society*, 17(3), 621–633. https://doi.org/10.1007/s10209-018-0609-5

Pew Research Center. (2018). *Social Media Use Continues to Rise in Developing Countries but Plateaus Across Developed Ones*. http://www.pewglobal.org/2018/06/19/2-smartphone-ownership-on-the-rise-in-emerging-economies/

Seifert, A., Hofer, M., & Rössel, J. (2018). Older adults' perceived sense of social exclusion from the digital world. *Educational Gerontology*, 44(12), 775–785. https://doi.org/10.1080/03601277.2019.1574415

Choosing Physical Distancing over Social Distancing in the Era of Technology: Minimizing Risk for Older People

Dear Editor,

Social distancing refers to a non-pharmaceutical intervention that is employed as a preventive measure to combat the spread of contagious diseases viz. COVID 19 by maintaining a safe distance between two individuals. However, the word 'safe distance' means a 'physical distance' rather than a 'social distance' (Abel & McQueen, 2020). Thus, the concept of social distancing covers conceptual as well as ethical aspects (Lewnard & Lo, 2020). Considering the practice of physical distancing, no two individuals must come within 6 feet of closeness (Centre for Disease Control & Prevention [CDC], 2020). It also enforces staying away from gatherings and crowded places. An important reason for adopting physical distancing as a measure is because we are unaware of the infected. An infected individual with COVID19 might be asymptomatic and during the latent phase he might be still able to communicate the disease to others. Therefore, the segregation of infected and non-infected becomes difficult. Moreover, the measure of physical distancing limits the scope of droplet transmission that is one of the major routes for COVID19. Older people are more susceptible to the disease as well as vulnerable to the psychological pressure.

Physical distancing poses a great problem to all sectors viz. academic, industry, production, etc., while the challenge lies highest within the aged/old population.

The fast pace of population aging around the world accounts to more than 900 million people of 60 years or more in 2015 (12% of population) and that is expected to grow to 22% of population by 2050 (WHO Fact Sheet, 2020). The participation of aged people is comparatively less in using online resources which results in problems of using online services like online-banking, tele-medicine, work-from-home, etc. (Reneland-Forsman, 2018). This also creates a lot of psychological fallout among older adults.

One of the best gifts of technology is to remain socially connected while maintaining physical distancing through social media like Whatsapp, Facebook, Twitter, Instagram, etc., as evidenced by their higher usage than normal situations (Warrington J, 2020). However, people are more habituated in meeting people physically, going to the bank, market, and public places rather than being confined to the mobile or laptop using social networking sites (Vroman et al., 2015). Therefore, the avenue of socializing is limited in such situations. The rural areas of various countries are also not well covered with network connectivity and usage largely depends on socio-economic conditions (Calvert et al., 2009).

Life expectancy of aged people is low in developing nations, which is further curtailed by epidemics like COVID 19 especially when old age serves as a risk factor.

Therefore, the optimal usage of technology along with medical and non-medical intervention can minimize the risk for aged people adhering to the rules of physical distancing while maintaining social connections, socio-economic disparity largely hinders the process.

Saptarshi Chatterjee

References

Abel, T., & McQueen, D. (2020). The COVID-19 pandemic calls for spatial distancing and social closeness: Not for social distancing! *International Journal of Public Health*, 65(3):231. https://doi.org/10.1007/s00038-020-01366-7

Calvert, J. F., Jr, Kaye, J., Leahy, M., Hexem, K., & Carlson, N. (2009). Technology use by rural and urban oldest old. *Technology and Health Care: Official Journal of the European Society for Engineering and Medicine*, 17(1), 1–11. https://doi.org/10.3233/THC-2009-0527

Centre for Disease Control & Prevention. (2020). National Center for Immunization and Respiratory Diseases (NCIRD), Division of Viral Diseases. https://www.cdc.gov/corona virus/2019-ncov/prevent-getting-sick/social-distancing.html

Coronavirus: 87% increase in social media usage amid lockdown; Indians spend 4 hours on Facebook, WhatsApp. Business Today. (Retrieved March 30, 2020, from https://www.busi nesstoday.in/technology/news/coronavirus-87-percent-increase-in-social-media-usage-amid-lockdown-indians-spend-4-hours-on-facebook-whatsapp/story/399571.html

Lewnard, J. A., & Lo, N. C. (2020). Scientific and ethical basis for social-distancing interventions against COVID-19. *The Lancet. Infectious Disease*. Advance online publication. https://doi.org/10.1016/S1473-3099(20)30190-0

Reneland-Forsman, L. (2018). 'Borrowed access' – The struggle of older persons for digital participation. *International Journal of Lifelong Education*, 37(3), 333–344. https://doi.org/10.1080/02601370.2018.1473516

Vroman, K. G., Arthanat, S., & Lysack, C. (2015). "Who over 65 is online?" Older adults' dispositions toward information communication technology. *Computers in Human Behavior*, 43[C], 156–166. https://doi.org/10.1016/j.chb.2014.10.018

Warrington, J. (2020, March 25). *Coronavirus: Whatsapp usage jumps 40 per cent during lockdown*. CITY A.M. From https://www.cityam.com/coronavirus-whatsapp-usage-jumps-40-per-cent-during-lockdown/

WHO-Fact sheet/Details/Aging & Health. (2020) https://www.who.int/news-room/fact-sheets/detail/ageing-and-health

Virtual Social Work Care with Older Black Adults: A Culturally Relevant Technology-Based Intervention to Reduce Social Isolation and Loneliness in a Time of Pandemic

Dear Editor,

The Public Health Agency of Canada, a federal agency of the Government of Canada, does not collect race-based data on COVID-19. Some provincial jurisdictions have begun collecting this information. From the limited data available, evidence shows a strong correlation between COVID-19 cases and neighborhoods with a higher number of Black people (Bowden & Cain, 2020).

Older Black adults are at an increased risk for COVID-19 for a number of reasons: poor socioeconomic status; living in rural/remote, high-density, or substandard physical environments; and difficulty accessing health care services (Bowden & Cain, 2020). Experience with anti-Black racism is also known to put members of Black and racialized communities at risk for COVID-19. These factors influence the health and social care of older Black adults, particularly those who are immunocompromised or present with underlying medical conditions, including diabetes, heart disease, hypertension, high blood pressure, and cancer.

In Canada, a clear disparity emerges in infection prevention and control measures to mitigate the impact of the pandemic on older Black adults, particularly those in rural or remote areas. Current measures for reducing the transmission of COVID-19 – including social distancing – do not take a racially and culturally informed approach to health and well-being. Racial stigma and privacy concerns may act as barriers to health care access for COVID-19 supportive care, and Black culture tends to prioritize collectivist over individualist values (Thabede, 2008) – multiple generations of family members may live in the same household. Family members who work in high-risk/low-wage jobs are at greater risk of contracting the disease, which can then spread to older family members.

Cultural institutions and places of worship are common sources of social support for older Black adults. In the context of COVID-19, connections fostered by these social networks are temporarily (or in the case of a death, permanently) severed. Older Black adults might experience feelings of isolation and loneliness due to public health measures that encourage social and physical distancing. Being isolated and lonely can exacerbate mental health conditions including anxiety, depression, and a decline in cognitive function or dementia (Fakoya et al., 2020).

Older Black adults in rural or remote areas could benefit from culturally responsive social work interventions that promote coping skills and social connections in periods of a public health crisis. *Virtual Social Work Care with Older Black Adults* is one such intervention strategy. This approach to gerontological care draws on an African epistemological and ontological world view (Thabede, 2008). Central to the model is the participation of older Black adults in their own social care within the supportive context of a virtual community.

In the proposed intervention strategy, as in the traditional African practice of Ubuntu, individuals would see themselves as part of a collective whole. Older Black adults would have a central role in identifying their own and the group's needs, and determine with social workers the best possible solution for meeting those needs. Even at a distance, the interdependent relationship between older Black adults and social workers would depart from the traditional Eurocentric social work practice where the practitioner holds power, determines what the service user needs, and prescribes individualistic solutions.

Culturally grounded interventions could support older Black adults to make new virtual connections that could reduce their social isolation and loneliness. Food is an important center of social interaction in Black culture. With support from a social worker, a digital meal could be organized, to engage older Black adults in sharing about their food and exchanging recipes. The prepared meals would then be eaten separately, at a distance, but simultaneously.

Positive religious coping and spirituality can have a beneficial impact on mental health and well-being (Koenig, 2009). Social workers could encourage dialogue among older Black adults about their immediate and future pandemic concerns, taking their religious and spiritual beliefs into consideration. Social workers could also help older Black adults maintain or improve their mobility, through regular group exercises combining playing African drums and dancing.

Ethical and legal challenges need to be considered in such a technology-based social intervention. Social workers must have open discussions with older Black adults about confidentiality when using communication technologies (Van Sickle, 2017). A security checklist for social workers and older Black adults – comprising encrypted devices, secure internet connections, and compliance with data privacy policies and standards – might minimize security vulnerabilities.

While the COVID-19 global pandemic has caused significant stress for older Black adults, particularly those who are socially and economically disadvantaged, social workers can take practical steps to minimize the negative consequences resulting from social and physical distancing measures. The holistic, virtual, and culturally sensitive intervention described here can help to reduce social isolation and loneliness as well as improve older Black adults' compliance with social and physical distancing guidelines.

Sincerely,

Sulaimon Giwa and Delores V. Mullings

ⓘ http://orcid.org/0000-0001-8076-0277

Karun K. Karki

References

Bowden, O., & Cain, P. (2020, June 2). *Black neighbourhoods in Toronto are hit hardest by COVID-19—and it's "anchored in racism": Experts.* Retrieved from https://globalnews.ca/news/7015522/black-neighbourhoods-toronto-coronavirus-racism/

Fakoya, O. A., McCorry, N. K., & Donnelly, M. (2020). Loneliness and social isolation interventions for older adults: A scoping review of reviews. *BMC Public Health, 20*(129). https://doi.org/10.1186/s12889-020-8251-6

Koenig, H. G. (2009). Research on religion, spirituality, and mental health: A review. *The Canadian Journal of Psychiatry, 54*(5), 283–291. https://doi.org/10.1177/070674370905400502

Thabede, D. (2008). The African worldview as the basis of practice in the helping professions. *Social Work/ Maatskaplike, 44*(3), 233–245.https://doi.org/10.15270/44-3-237

Van Sickle, C. (2017). *Practice notes: Professional and ethical communication technology practices and policies for a digital world.* Retrieved from https://perspective.ocswssw.org/practice-notes-professional-and-ethical/

Social Responses for Older People in COVID-19 Pandemic: Experience from Vietnam

Dear Editor,

For a few months, a novel coronavirus disease (COVID-19) has spread globally. The World Health Organization has been coordinating the global efforts to control the negative effects and announced COVID-19 as a global pandemic in March 2020. Particularly, on April 20, 2020, there were nearly 2.4 million confirmed cases and nearly 165 thousand deaths (Worldometers, 2020). The negative effect of this epidemic was unprecedented when about 20% of the global population (nearly 1.7 billion people) must work from home and many countries had to enter lockdown to fight the disease (Davidson, 2020; Gopinath, 2020). It is also emphasized that COVID-19 pandemic is the biggest threat to the whole of humanity since the Second World War with unprecedented risks (United Nations, 2020). Many urgent solutions have been applied by many countries to slow down the spread of this dangerous disease (Lee & Morling, 2020), however, the current situation is still very serious (United Nations, 2020).

According to the World Health Organization, the COVID-19 pandemic is affecting the global population in drastic ways, however, older people are facing the most threats and challenges at this time. Especially in areas with high rates of older people, 95% of death cases those older than 60 years (World Health Organization, 2020). In Vietnam, older people are defined as persons aged 60 and over (Ministry of Health, 2017). The aging population is a social challenge in Vietnam now (Figure 1). This country will be one of the rapidly aging countries in the world in the next 30 years (Giang et al., 2019).

The statistical report pointed out that the aging of the population in Vietnam has occurred quickly with the population aged 60 years and older is 11.3 million people (accounting for about 11.7% of the total population). The Vietnamese aging index was 48.8% in 2019, an increase of 13.3% points compared to 2009 and twice as much as 1999 (General Statistics Office of Vietnam, 2019). According to data from the Ministry of Health, the Vietnamese people aged 60 years and older have 2.6 diseases on average, besides, the population aged 80 years and older have 6.8 on average (Ministry of Health, 2017). Like many Asian countries, the older people in Vietnam often live with later generations in a large family. In the same situation as many countries in the COVID-19 pandemic, Vietnam is carefully protecting older people now.

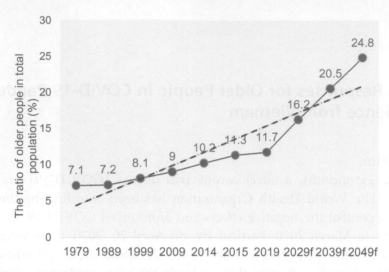

Figure 1. The ratio of Vietnamese older people in total population, 1979–2049. Source: Ministry of Health (2017).

In the context of the COVID-19 outbreak rapidly around the world, Vietnam is becoming a highlighted country that is successfully coping with the risk of the virus spreading in society (Fleming, 2020; Reed, 2020). In fact, Vietnam has high risks from COVID-19 because this country has a quite large population of nearly 97 million people (ranked 15th in the world), the series virus outbreak of neighbor countries, and its high economic openness. However, the success of Vietnam is proved by the very low rate of positive cases (as 0.0002% of the population) and still no-death (Worldometers, 2020). Until 22/04/2020, there are 80% of patients recovered in the total number of 268 confirmed cases (Ministry of Health, 2020). The Vietnamese government is said to have taken reasonable and timely responses to deal with the COVID-19 pandemic, besides, the people are also highly appreciated for the compliance level as well as their trust and support for the government activities (Ebbighausen, 2020; Sullivan, 2020). In addition, the good experiences gained from being the first successful country in dealing with the SARS epidemic (in 2003) also have brought much value to Vietnam in the current situation. The urgent and strong activities of the government, socio-political organizations, entrepreneurs and private sponsors and a high consensus of the people have helped Vietnam to contain the spread of disease.

The descriptive statistics (Figure 2) show that the number of older patients is the smallest in the sample of 218 COVID-19 confirmed cases (accounting for only 10% of the total number of patients). Although there are some older patients having diseases, there is still no-death due to COVID-19 in Vietnam. This is in contrast to the situation in most other countries because a large number of Vietnamese patients are young people (20–29 years), accounting for 37% because they were the Vietnamese returning (education or labor

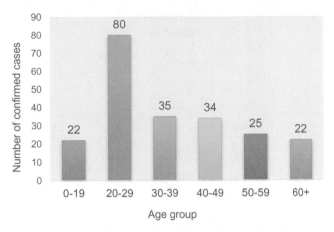

Figure 2. Distribution of age among 218 COVID-19 patients in Vietnam. Source: Ministry of Health (2020).

targets) from countries with outbreaks of disease. At the beginning of February 2020, the government closed schools which helped to limit the spread of COVID-19 to children and young people. The number of older infections in Vietnam is very small compared to other countries. Against the risks of disease outbreaks, in order to protect the older people, the most vulnerable group with COVID-19, the Ministry of Health and socio-political organizations have continuously suggested older people need to stay home and practice the social distaining solution (Government, 2020). In some big cities (eg., in Ho Chi Minh City), doctors and nurses come to examine at home and promote online medical advice for older patients.

In the COVID-19 pandemic, Vietnamese older people have received much interest as the most vulnerable and at-risk from the virus. There have been diverse social responses for older people in the fight the COVID-19 outbreak in Vietnam including actions of the government, socio-political organizations, entrepreneurs and private sponsors. Since the first infection case was reported, there were some strong slogans including "Fighting against epidemic like fighting against an enemy" and "No one was left behind in the fight against COVID-19" announced by the government. Because of many efficient activities, unlike many other countries in the world, there is only 10% of COVID-19 patients are older people in Vietnam. Success in preventing the infection of older people is also part of the overall success of fighting against this disease in Vietnam (Pangescu, 2020).

A coordinated social response is extremely important to successfully contain a dangerous pandemic such as COVID-19. As shown in Figure 3, there are three main responses from society to the older people in Vietnam, including the responses of the government, social-political organizations, entrepreneurs and private sponsors. This model can be explained in more detail below.

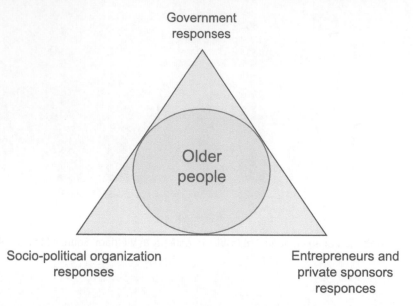

Figure 3. The model of social responses for older people in COVID-19 pandemic in Vietnam. Source: Author's elaboration.

The Vietnamese government responses are very efficient with short and strong emergency slogans to directly express to people, especially disadvantaged older people. The COVID-19 pandemic is urgently informed by a variety of information channels such as mobile-phone messages, social media networks (e.g., Facebook, Youtube, and Zalo), television, newspapers, and radio. The government developed websites to monitor the traveling history of citizens. There were some public policies issued to support disadvantaged groups negatively affected by the COVID-19 pandemic. Older people receive benefits (like all people) in free testing, free isolation, and free medical treatment. In blockaded areas, people are provided free foods during the time of isolation (e.g., Truc Bach ward in Hanoi). Some subsidies have been implemented such as direct cash payments and free essential foods. The Ministry of Health issued two documents guidelines regarding "Health management of the elderly group and people with chronic diseases in the context of an epidemic COVID-19" and "A guide to healthcare for preventing and fighting COVID-19 for the elderly in the community". The national social security organization paid pensions and benefits for older people at their homes. The home health care program for the elderly group is performed in some provinces (for example, in Ho Chi Minh City).

Socio-political organizations have an important role to launch charitable and voluntary movements in caring for and supporting vulnerable people (for example, lonely older people). The Fatherland Front establishes charity funds to help with the prevention and control of the COVID-19 pandemic. Youth Union provides free foods for the lonely elderly people and the disadvantaged people in some provinces and supports propaganda to households the good ways to prevent COVID-19. The Women Union gives essential foods to lonely elderly women in society.

There are many activities from entrepreneurs and private sponsors to support the disadvantaged people who have been negatively affected by COVID-19. The financial resource is funding by entrepreneurs and private donors in Vietnam. For example, the construction of equipment such as 'rice ATM' to distribute rice for free to vulnerable people in many provinces (Duong, 2020). At some charitable places, besides rice, eggs and vegetables are freely distributed to the poor people.

The effective model for combating the COVID-19 pandemic in Vietnam is a successful example in the current context. With many strong and multi-dimensional solutions, Vietnam has maintained a low number of confirmed infections as well as a very small number of older patients. My paper presents a model that helps Vietnam not only prevent the spread of the COVID-19 but also ensure social security for older people (and vulnerable people in general). As a country with a high aging population, the Vietnamese social response model is built as a comprehensive platform efficiency merging the activities of many directions including the government, socio-political organizations, entrepreneurs, and private sponsors. Vietnam provides a good practice model for other countries (especially the countries that have limited resources) in order to successfully cope with the ongoing impacts of the COVID-19 pandemic.

Le Thanh Tung

References

Davidson, H. (2020, April 15). Around 20% of global population under coronavirus lockdown. *Theguardian.com*. https://www.theguardian.com/world/2020/mar/24/nearly-20-of-global-population-under-coronavirus-lockdown

Duong, Y. (2020, April 20). 'Rice ATM' feeds Vietnam's poor amid virus lockdown. *Reuters.com*. https://www.reuters.com/article/us-health-coronavirus-vietnam-riceatm/rice-atm-feeds-vietnams-poor-amid-virus-lockdown-idUSKCN21V0GQ

Ebbighausen, R. (2020, April 20). How Vietnam is winning its 'war' on coronavirus. *Deutsche Welle*. https://www.dw.com/en/how-vietnam-is-winning-its-war-on-coronavirus/a-52929967

Fleming, S. (2020). *Viet Nam shows how you can contain COVID-19 with limited resources*. World Economic Forum. https://www.weforum.org/agenda/2020/03/vietnam-contain-covid-19-limited-resources/

General Statistics Office of Vietnam. (2019). *The Vietnam population and housing census Statistical Publishing House, Hanoi*, Vietnam.

Giang, T. L., Nguyen, N. T., Nguyen, T. T., Le, H. Q., & Tran, N. T. T. (2020). Social support effect on health of older people in Vietnam: Evidence from a national aging survey. *Ageing International.* https://doi.org/10.1007/s12126-020-09370-1

Gopinath, G. (2020). *The great lockdown: Worst economic downturn since the great depression.* International Monetary Fund. https://blogs.imf.org/2020/04/14/the-great-lockdown-worst-economic-downturn-since-the-great-depression/

Government. (2020, April 21). Online newspapers of the Government, Vietnam. http://www.chinhphu.vn/portal/page/portal/chinhphu/trangchu/lanhdaochidao

Lee, A., & Morling, J. (2020). COVID19 - The need for public health in a time of emergency. *Public Health, 182*(5), 188–189. https://doi.org/10.1016/j.puhe.2020.03.027

Ministry of Health. (2017). *Joint annual health review 2016: Towards healthy aging in Vietnam (JAHR2016_Edraft).* http://jahr.org.vn/downloads/JAHR2016/JAHR2016_Edraft.pdf

Ministry of Health. (2020, April 22). COVID-19 information page. https://ncov.moh.gov.vn/

Pangescu, M. E. (2020). *For the poorest countries, the full danger from Corona virus is only just coming into view.* World Bank. https://blogs.worldbank.org/voices/poorest-countries-full-danger-coronavirus-only-just-coming-view

Reed, J. (2020). Vietnam's coronavirus offensive wins praise for low-cost model. *Financial Times.* https://www.ft.com/content/0cc3c956-6cb2-11ea-89df-41bea055720b

Sullivan, M. (2020, April 18). In Vietnam, there have been fewer than 200 COVID-19 cases and no deaths. Here's why. *Npr.com.* https://www.npr.org/sections/coronavirus-live-updates/2020/04/16/835748673/in-vietnam-there-have-been-fewer-than-300-covid-19-cases-and-no-deaths-heres-why

United Nations (2020, April 15). Launch of Global humanitarian response plan for COVID-19. https://www.un.org/sg/en/content/sg/press-encounter/2020-03-25/launch-of-global-humanitarian-response-plan-for-covid-19

World Health Organization (2020, April 18). Older people are at highest risk from COVID-19 - the evidence and solutions. http://www.euro.who.int/en/health-topics/health-emergencies/coronavirus-covid-19/news/news/2020/4/supporting-older-people-during-the-covid-19-pandemic-is-everyones-business

Worldometers. (2020, April 20). Conona virus update. https://www.worldometers.info/coronavirus/

Fighting COVID-19: Fear and Internal Conflict among Older Adults in Ghana

Dear Editor,

Upon the World Health Organization's declaration as a *Public Health Emergency of International Concern* (WHO, 2020), the novel coronavirus has taken a global tour and Africa is envisaged as the next epicenter of the infection. Ghana's first two cases of COVID-19 were confirmed on 12 March 2020. These individuals had returned to Ghana from Norway and Turkey and a few days later became ill. After these index cases, Ministry of Health deployed mechanisms to scale-up contact tracing and tesing for potential cases. The number of COVID-19 confirmed cases have been increasing exponentially over the past two months (5735 case and 29 deaths as of 17 May 2020), and these are perhaps substantial underestimates (Ghana Health Service, 2020).

Like the global situation, it is highly melancholic that older adults 60 years or over in Ghana have faced higher infection and mortality rates compared to the general population. The trends are even gloomy for those with comorbidities such as cardiovascular diseases, chronic respiratory disease, active cancers, and diabetes (Kang et al., 2020). The mortality rate of COVID-19 is 15% for older people 80 years or over compared to 0.2% for those under 20 years (Worldometer, 2020a). Age is, therefore, a critical variable posing a major risk for COVID-19 mortality and has created serious emotional disturbances and insecurity and major anxiety and depressive disorders among older people. At the same time, these vulnerable older people are being imperiled with ageism in the thoughts and discourse of the public. They face neglect and experience domestic abuse at home and also suffer age discriminations even in health care access and use. These circumstances present crucial implications for social policies, public health, and clinical response particularly in resource constrained countries such as Ghana.

Given the heightened public health burden of COVID-19, the Government of Ghana (GoG) like many other political leaders in Africa implemented interventions to prevent the potential importation and subsequent community spread of the virus. On 30 March 2020, the GoG announced closure of borders and partial lockdown in the hotspots of COVID-19 infections. The GoG also placed a nationwide ban on social gathering by closing down educational institutions, religious activities and provided stringent directives on the use of public transport. Like many low-income settings, lockdown and the concomitant social and physical distancing deepen poverty and hunger particularly among the poor in Ghana. It also stimulated a sudden separation of older people from loved ones, casused a shortage of living supplies, loss of freedom, and uncertainty over disease status.

On 19 April 2020, the GoG indicated a *lift* of the lockdown regulations instituted to enhance physical and social distancing protocols. At the same time, COVID-19 cases in the country had been skyrocketing, placing Ghana at the fifth position in the continent (after South Africa, Egypt, Morocco, and Algeria) (Worldometer, 2020b). Whilst many have described the action of GoG as premature, others contend that it is a way to reduce hardships associated with lockdown and restrictions on movement. The Director-General of WHO, Dr Tedros Adhanom Ghebreyesus warned all countries that Coronavirus could re-surge if the lockdown restrictions are lifted too early. Gilbert et al. (2020) have earlier cautioned that the ability of Ghana and other African countries to manage community spread of the virus after importation will depend upon the application of stern measures of detection, prevention, and control. These scuffles caused serious "moral panic" engulfed with fear and aggravated anxiety and psychological insecurity among the at-risk older people, creating a deleterious impacts on their mental health and quality of life.

Now that COVID-19 has no vaccine or standardized treatment modality, a critical question remains, that would Ghana's health system be able to contain the alarming cases of COVID-19 and adjust appropriately to deal with the specific needs of older people? Like many countries in the continent, the capacity of Ghana to provide sufficient infrastructure, personnel, and clinical care to support those who will test positive through the local cycles of transmission of COVID-19 has been questioned vehemently and declared highly vulnerable (Gilbert et al., 2020).

The considerations and modalities to fight COVID-19 should be backed by *science* and not mere speculations. Effectively translating and incorporating data and science into both operational and policy action should be a universal priority. I strongly propose that the health system should be realigned and prepare for a geriatric care and support for older people who are highly at-risk of the pandemic. Moreover, a complete enforcement of stringent preventive measures such as *mandatory* use of facial masks in public places will be golden to stop the spread of COVID-19 especially to older people. Besides, culturally oriented educational interventions and platforms for psychological counseling services and care for older adults in general as well as COVID-19 infected, at-risk and affected populations specifically will increase public understanding and also safeguard mental health of those vulnerable to the pandemic. A multi-sectoral synergies are urgently needed to effectively address the huge impact of COVID-19 in Ghana particularly among older adults. We cannot afford to ignore older adults especially those with non-communicable diseases in the fight against COVID-19.

Sincerely,

Razak M Gyasi

iD http://orcid.org/0000-6733-1539

References

Ghana Health Service. (2020). *Situation update, confirmed Covid-19 cases in Ghana as at 25 April 2020, 22:00hrs. COVID-19: Ghana's outbreak response management updates.*, Ghana Health Service and Ministry of Health. https://ghanahealthservice.org/covid19/

Gilbert, M., Pullano, G., Pinotti, F., Valdano, E., Poletto, C., Boëlle, P.-Y., D'Ortenzio, E., Yazdanpanah, Y., Eholie, S. P., Altmann, M., Gutierrez, B., Kraemer, M. U. G., & Colizza, V. (2020). Preparedness and vulnerability of African countries against importations of COVID-19: A modelling study. *The Lancet*, *395*(10227), 871–877. https://doi.org/10.1016/S0140–6736(20)30411–6

Kang, C., Yang, S., Yuan, J., Xu, L., Zhao, X., & Yang, J. (2020). Patients with chronic illness urgently need integrated physical and psychological care during the COVID-19 outbreak. *Asian Journal of Psychiatry*, *51*, 102081. https://doi.org/10.1016/j.ajp.2020.102081

WHO. (2020). *WHO Emergency Committee Statement on the second meeting of the International Health Regulations, 2005. Emergency Committee regarding the outbreak of novel coronavirus (COVID-19).* The World Health Organization, Geneva. https://www.who.int/news-room/detail/30-01-2020-statement-on-the-second-meeting-of-the-international-health-regulations-(2005)-emergency-committee-regarding-the-outbreak-of-novel-coronavirus-(COVID-19)

Worldometer. (2020a). *Age, sex, existing conditions of COVID-19 cases and deaths.* The World Health Organization, Geneva. Retrieved April, 25, 2020, from https://www.worldometers.info/coronavirus/coronavirus-age-sex-demographics/

Worldometer. (2020b). *Countries where COVID-19 has spread.* The World Health Organization, Geneva. Retrieved April, 25, 2020, from https://www.worldometers.info/coronavirus/countries-where-coronavirus-has-spread/

Re-integrating Older Adults Who Have Recovered from the Novel Coronavirus into Society in the Context of Stigmatization: Lessons for Health and Social Actors in Ghana

Dear Editor,

The novel coronavirus (COVID-19) was first identified in Wuhan, China in December 2019 and has become one of the most serious public health crisis in the world. People, especially the vulnerable populations such as older adults and those with underlying health conditions continue to struggle with the virus (Jung & Jun, 2020; Bruns et al., 2020; World Health Organization [WHO], 2020a; Arthur-Holmes & Agyemang-Duah, 2020). One major social consequence of contracting the deadly virus is the stigmatization of COVID-19 patients, including older adults. In view of this, we write to offer lessons for health and social actors on how to re-integrate older adults who have recovered from the COVID-19 infection into society in the context of stigmatization.

Pronounced stigmatization among COVID-19 patients, including those who have recovered stems from three overlapping factors. First, the disease is new and for that matter there are still many unknowns. Second, people are often afraid of the unknown. Third, it is easy to associate that fear with other people (WHO, 2020b). Thus, knowledge gaps in connection with the COVID-19 infection are likely to result in stigmatization. However, stigmatization prevents people from either testing for the virus or seeking immediate healthcare when they experience symptoms of the COVID-19 infection (Bruns et al., 2020).

Owing to the counterproductive nature of stigmatization in the management and containment of COVID-19, concerted stakeholder actions are required to address this social issue. First, to the health actors, we recommend the development of a comprehensive plan for dealing with the stigmatization to ensure a successful re-integration of older adults who have recovered from the COVID-19 infection into society. Further, policy and social actors should push for the passage of appropriate regulations and laws that will make stigmatization of patients, including older adults who have recovered from the COVID-19 infection a punishable and prosecutable offense. Moreover, public health stakeholders and social workers should make an effort to integrate anti-stigma measures into public health and social work education to prevent stigmatization .

Specifically, public health actors and social workers should organize frequent meetings, fora, workshops, and conferences on radios and televisions for sensitization of community members on the consequences of stigmatization. Besides, as a way of ensuring that the rights of older adults who have recovered from the COVID-19 infection are protected, efforts must be made to shield their identities . These policy measures are therefore critical in our quest to successfully re-integrate older adults who have recovered from the COVID-19 infection into society in the context of stigmatization.   Sincerely,

Williams Agyemang-Duah

ⓘ http://orcid.org/0000-0001-
8658-004X
Anthony Kwame Morgan

ⓘ http://orcid.org/0000-0001-7904-9955
Joseph Oduro Appiah

ⓘ http://orcid.org/0000-0001-9370-4004
Prince Peprah

ⓘ http://orcid.org/0000-0002-3816-2713
Audrey Amponsah Fordjour

References

Arthur-Holmes, F., & Agyemang-Duah, W. (2020). Reaching older adults during the COVID-19 pandemic through social networks and Social Security Schemes in Ghana: Lessons for considerations. Journal of Gerontological Social Work, 1-3. doi:doi.10.1080/01634372.2020.1764689

Bruns, D. P., Kraguljac, N. V., & Bruns, T. R. (2020). Covid-19: Facts, cultural considerations, and risk of stigmatization. *Journal of Transcultural Nursing, 31*(4), 326-332.

Jung, S. J., & Jun, J. Y. (2020). Mental health and psychological intervention amid COVID-19 outbreak: Perspectives from South Korea. *Yonsei Medical Journal, 61*(4), 271–272. https://doi.org/10.3349/ymj.2020.61.4.271

World Economic Forum (2020b). *Social Stigma associated with COVID-19*. Accessed from https://www.who.int/docs/default-source/coronaviruse/covid19-stigma-guide.pdf, on 20 May 2020

World Health Organization [WHO]. (2020a). *Coronavirus disease (COVID19) pandemic*. Retrieved April 25, 2020, from https://www.who.int/emergencies/diseases/novel-coronavirus-2019/

Part VI

Interventions to Support Older Adults during COVID-19

Staying Isolated in Order to Stay Safe: Exploring Experiences of the MIT AgeLab 85+ Lifestyle Leaders during the COVID-19 Pandemic

Dear Editor,

In a special issue of the *Journal of Gerontological Social Work* on disaster preparedness, Kusmaul et al. (2018) explained that one role of gerontological social workers in disaster preparedness and response is to identify unique needs, risk factors, and strengths possessed by older adults during periods of disaster. We would like to describe how a developing study of ours strives to understand these characteristics as they pertain to the "oldest old" – that is, adults ages 85 and over – in the midst of the disaster spurred by the current global spread of COVID-19.

While chronological age does not solely determine risk of falling ill or dying from COVID-19, a combination of physiological and social/structural factors render the "oldest old" more vulnerable in general (Centers for Disease Control and Prevention, 2020). There is much to be learned about how the "oldest old" – particularly those who are relatively healthy and active – are faring during this time of physical distancing.

Since 2015, the MIT AgeLab has convened a bimonthly research panel of adults ages 85 and older called the 85+ Lifestyle Leaders panel. Beginning in March 2020, we engaged the Lifestyle Leaders in mixed-methods research about their experiences during COVID-19. We fielded an online survey in mid-March and have continued to follow up with a longitudinal diary study. Data collection is still underway, with over twenty weekly phone interviews and activity tracking having been conducted so far.

One observation we have already is the resilience of the Lifestyle Leaders in managing the negative effects of physical distancing. In ordinary circumstances, physical distancing (and its byproducts, social isolation and loneliness) would be treated as a risk factor for older adults, not as a protective measure (Holt-Lunstad et al., 2015). However, with many Lifestyle Leaders accustomed to some forms of social and physical distance already, life for many of them during the pandemic, especially those with more limited mobility, is largely business-as-usual. Given this potential advantage in adapting to social and physical distancing, the Lifestyle Leaders may be specially equipped to offer advice for staying healthy and connected during an undetermined period of isolation.

A second early insight is that many Lifestyle Leaders have described a loss of control that – while surely endemic across all age groups during the pandemic – surfaces in unique ways for the 85+ population. The unpredictable progression of government regulation restricting everyone's daily activities is mirrored by the rapid implementation of regulations within age-restricted group living environments that many of the Lifestyle Leaders inhabit. Uncertainty and anxiety loom in the background for many Lifestyle Leaders due to other factors as well, such as food scarcity, not knowing where to turn for help should they need it, and a heightened sense of mortality and vulnerability due to the spread of an invisible killer.

Based on our preliminary findings, we suggest social workers can help the "oldest old" combat feelings of helplessness or helplessness as a result of COVID-19 in a variety of ways:

- Offering instrumental support to ensure those facing scarcity have their basic needs met. Particularly for those with limited mobility or without loved ones nearby, social workers can connect older adults with home delivery resources to assist them.
- Reinforcing older adults' sense of purpose and agency when they may otherwise be made to feel helpless. Social workers can support older adults' determination of how they desire to stay occupied, including sharing flexible volunteer opportunities that can be done virtually, over the phone, or in another kind of physically distanced way.
- Empowering older adults' sense of technological industry. The frustrations experienced by digital nonnatives toward technology are amplified during a stressful and abruptly device-dependent time. Physical distancing means many of our Lifestyle Leaders, including those who would self-identify as "less tech-savvy," are engaging (and often struggling alone) with devices that are their only connection to the outside world. Social workers can help older adults access technologies that are increasingly lifelines for many, including those 85 and over – to get information, to socialize, and even to meet basic needs.

The challenges of COVID-19 are unique but not unlike other trials the Lifestyle Leaders have overcome in their lifetimes. We look forward to learning more from the 85+ Lifestyle Leaders with the ultimate goal of building on Kusmaul et al.'s (2018) guidance for gerontological social workers involved in disaster preparedness and response.

Julie B. Miller and Taylor R. Patskanick and Lisa A. D'Ambrosio and Joseph F. Coughlin

(ID) http://orcid.org/0000-0003-2129-5074

References

Centers for Disease Control and Prevention. (2020). *Coronavirus disease 2019 (COVID-19): Older adults.* https://www.cdc.gov/coronavirus/2019-ncov/need-extra-precautions/older-adults.html

Holt-Lunstad, J., Smith, T. B., Baker, M., Harris, T., & Stephenson, D. (2015). Loneliness and social isolation as risk factors for mortality: A meta-analytic review. *Perspectives on Psychological Science, 10* (2), 227–237. https://doi.org/10.1177/1745691614568352

Kusmaul, N., Gibson, A., & Leedahl, S. N. (2018). Gerontological social work roles in disaster preparedness and response. *Journal of Gerontological Social Work, 61*(7), 692–696. https://doi.org/10.1080/01634372.2018.1510455

Adapting 'Sunshine,' A Socially Assistive Chat Robot for Older Adults with Cognitive Impairment: A Pilot Study

Dear Editor,

During the COVID-19 pandemic, older adults with cognitive impairment in long-term care facilities, who are already excluded from much of social life, have been asked to distance themselves even further, deepening their loneliness. Many have died alone, separated from their family and friends. As we chart untested waters in gerontological social work, we must think outside of the box to respond to this unprecedented global crisis. A Socially Assistive Robot (SAR) is our example of such thinking.

SARs have potential to help seniors (Abdi et al., 2018). Advances in speech recognition and natural language processing provide more humanlike robots that offer cognitive assistance, social interaction, and stimulating activities. Conversational interaction is especially important: older residents with Alzheimer's Disease and related dementia (ADRD) have limited opportunity to chat, sing, or play simple games unless family members/friends come to visit.

We are currently designing and implementing a study to evaluate usability and acceptability of a SAR by eliciting perspectives of older adults with ADRD who interact with it. Our project uses "Sunshine," a Korean-manufactured, English-speaking doll-chatbot system. The 30-inch doll simulates a 7-year old grandchild, incorporating body/costume sensors and AI features for talk. Its small, soft body allows people to hold, snuggle, and converse with it: see https://youtu.be/rsugACFsRl0 (Studio CrossCulture, 2020).

Sunshine can be programed to remind users of meals, medications, and appointments. It can play songs, cue reminiscences, quote inspirational passages, tell stories, and play Simon Says. Sunshine's conversations encourage exercise and social engagement, functioning as a stress reliever to calm agitation and may elicit speech from previously unresponsive residents. Sunshine has decreased geriatric depression and improved quality of sleep and cognition among older patients living alone in South Korea (Kim et al., in press). Its efficacy needs testing in real-life U.S. situations for persons with ADRD and their care partners.

Our pilot (1) investigates whether assistive and social characteristics of a cuddly Sunshine-doll can motivate older adults with ADRD to engage in conversational interaction and other activities, enhancing quality of life; and (2) assesses barriers and facilitators to using telehealth for research with residents and caregivers.

For this pilot, 30 participants, aged 60-plus and diagnosed with ADRD will be recruited from adult care and nursing homes in our area with special attention paid to recruiting from all genders and diverse races. Informed consent will be obtained from all guardians and caregivers and assent will be obtained from participants in keeping with appropriate Human Subjects Review (IRB) guidelines. As of this writing, we are in the final stage of establishing IRB protocols and obtaining letters of support.

This study has three phases: pre-intervention, intervention, and post-intervention interactions. Phase 1 introduces Sunshine, using teleconferencing for discussions of whether residents might see Sunshine as beneficial and what it might be like to keep Sunshine (Chu et al., 2017). Telehealth (videoconferencing and e-mobile apps) will deliver training in Sunshine's use to participants and facility caregivers.

In phase 2, the researchers will rent each participant a Sunshine doll for up to three months during the study period. Caregivers (and research assistants once visitors are allowed) will use teleconferencing and e-mobile phones to video–record interactions.

In phase 3, each participant is invited to individual conversations with a research team member (teleconferencing or face-to-face) to discuss their experiences and thoughts about Sunshine. We will ask questions using an empathetic style and brief follow-up probes (Cridland et al., 2016): what participants liked or disliked about Sunshine; what they wanted to change.

This intervention's strength is the flexibility in its service delivery. Since remote technology is already customized into Sunshine, it can be easily integrated into usual care practices, using only existing staff and resources. Participants and caregivers are instructed on how to turn Sunshine on and off, but users are free to choose how and when to interact. They will be asked not to sleep or bathe with it (for safety reasons), nor to take it out of the home (to prevent loss).

Outcomes for 30 participants will be measured pre- and post-intervention by administration of standardized scales, either in person and/or through teleconferencing. The primary predicted clinical outcome will be reduction of apathy, delirium, and cognitive disorders for residents, measured by the Global Deterioration Scale and Apathy Inventory. Secondary outcomes should include the expansion of conversational and interpersonal interaction stimulated by using Sunshine. Perceptions by caregivers of resident interactions are assessed with the Dementia Quality of Life Scale for Proxy Caregivers. They will be asked privately for reflections about using SAR dolls. Qualitative discourse analyses of data will follow Jones et al. (2015) to combine behavioral ratings with video of robot–human partnerships.

Sunshine's sensors present an easy, robust way to collect data from constant motion detection in response to personalized voice reminders for medication, exercise, and interactions around stories and music. Sensors will communicate with data collection and management services through Web Application Interface. Data collected will be analyzed to build learning models to detect different user actions and engagement.

Thinking outside of the box requires new partnerships and skills. In light of the COVID-19 pandemic, we must come up with bold and innovative ways to deliver services for socially isolated persons with ADRD and their care partners: Sunshine SAR exemplifies our bold strategy. Findings will be used to develop and seek funding for a larger trial.

Othelia EunKyoung Lee

Boyd Davis

References

Abdi, J., Al-Hindawi, A., Ng, T., & Vizcaychipi, M. (2018). Scoping review on the use of socially assistive robot technology in elderly care. *BMJ Open*, *8*(2), e018815. https://doi.org/10.1136/bmjopen-2017-018815

Chu, M., Khosla, R., Mohammad, S., Khaksar, S., & Nguyen, K. (2017). Service innovation through social robot engagement to improve dementia care quality. *Assistive Technology*, *29*(1), 8–18. https://doi.org/10.1080/10400435.2016.1171807

Cridland, E., Phillipson, L., Brennan-Horley, C., & Swaffer, K. (2016). Reflections and recommendations for conducting in-depth interviews with people with dementia. *Qualitative Health Research*, *26*(13), 1–9. https://doi.org/10.1177/1049732316637065

Jones, C., Sung, B., & Moyle, W. (2015). Assessing engagement in people with dementia: A new approach to assessment using video analysis. *Archives. Psychiatric Nursing.*, *29*(6), 377–382. https://doi.org/10.1016/j.apnu.2015.06.019

Kim, Y., Lee, H., Kim, T., Kim, J., & Ok, K. (in press). The effect of care-robots on improving anxiety/depression and drug compliance among the elderly in the community. *Korean Medical Research Journal*.

Studio CrossCulture. (2020). *Sunshine's function*. https://youtu.be/rsugACFsRl0.

Reaching older adults during the COVID-19 pandemic through social networks and Social Security Schemes in Ghana: Lessons for considerations

Dear Editor,

The lives of older people are at risk during the COVID-19 pandemic as their immune system is weak to fight the virus. It has been reported that older people are more susceptible to COVID-19 and have higher likelihood of dying from the disease (Heymann & Shindo, 2020; Kinner et al., 2020). Like many other low- and middle-income countries (LMICs), Ghana may find it difficult to provide financial resources as a relief package to older people during the pandemic to reduce its impact on their lives. Therefore, we write to offer options on how older adults can be supported through social networks and social security schemes in Ghana during this pandemic.

As some governments of the developed countries began to provide relief packages and made promises to their citizens, the developing countries, especially those in the sub-Saharan Africa have followed their footsteps. For instance, the UK government has pledged to pay wage subsidies of 80% for salaried workers for some months to avoid layoffs and has also informed self-employed people that they can apply for a grant worth 80% of their average monthly profits over the last 3 years (Islam, 2020). In the United States, a sum of 2 USD trillion stimulus package has been announced with direct payments of up to 1200 USD to individuals (Rein, 2020). In Ghana, the government has decided to fully absorb electricity bills of all Ghanaians for 3 months from Aprilto June, particularly those who consume 0–50 kilowatt-hours a month for this period. In an effort to fight against the COVID-19 as most countries which reported cases of the virus have done, the government of Ghana placed some parts of the country – Greater Accra and Greater Kumasi Metropolitan Area– under 3-week lockdown including the one week lockdown extension (from 30 March to 19 April 2020) after recording 152 cases of COVID-19. Before the 3 week partial lockdown, the government established the COVID-19 National Trust Fund to fight the disease.

In the Ghanaian society, family is the core of its structure. However, the role of each member in the family goes beyond his/her place within it or a sense of belonging. Every member has a responsibility of ensuring that the welfare of other members is met. During the lockdown, social support networks and some social organisations helped older people in the lockdown areas to survive through the provision of foodstuffs and meals. That notwithstanding, some social workers also played a crucial role in educating Ghanaians about their responsibilities in the fight against COVID-19 and observing social distancing measures.

More is therefore required from social protection agencies in educating the older population on COVID-19 and its preventive measures. This is as a result of the misinformation and disinformation on the pandemic among the general Ghanaian population. Although the government has lifted the lockdown in the Greater Kumasi Metropolitan Area and parts of Greater Accra Region, there is still the need for social protection agencies and family heads to "step up" and provide support to older people to improve their quality of lives during the pandemic. This support should therefore come from different forms including advice, emotional, financial, and material. In these difficult times, physical movement support appears to be difficult as the preventive measures to fight the disease disallow physical contact. It is important to note that older people may still need to utilize their social networks through their friends, relatives, neighbors, and social organizations (such as religious organizations) in order to meet their basic needs. Hence, the existing relationship between older people and their social support networks needs to be strengthened. Since social distancing and isolation come with their own risks, social protection agencies and family heads or members should encourage older people to stay at home and learn how to use social media to entertain themselves in order to avoid loneliness and mental health problems.

It is worth noting that Ghana's economy is predominantly informal which makes it difficult for people to secure their future through pension schemes. Many older people depend on their children as a social security in later life. As a consequence, when their children lose their source of livelihood, their support services and income inflow become affected, which subsequently increases their vulnerability. Employed and unemployed older people aged 50+, who are financially and economically affected by the pandemic, may need support social protection from social institutions, particularly the Social Security and National Insurance Trust (SSNIT). It is therefore crucial for SSNIT and financial institutions to make provisions for these affected older people to receive portion of their pension package to meet their basic needs during the pandemic.

In addition, government should release the Livelihood Empowerment against Poverty Programme bi-monthly funds on time to the beneficiaries' older people. Considering the fact that the funds are inadequate to cater for the needs of older people with very low incomes, government should make an effort to increase the amount temporary (3 months) amidst the COVID-19 pandemic. Also, the non-governmental organizations that are into social protection should make an effort to provide social support to older people to improve their living conditions. During this pandemic, social interventions are critical in improving the quality of lives of older adults in Ghana.

Sincerely,

Francis Arthur-Holmes

http://orcid.org/0000-0002-5099-4555

Williams Agyemang-Duah

http://orcid.org/0000-0001-8658-004X

References

BBC News. (2020, March 26). *Coronavirus: UK government unveils aid for self employed.* Retrieved April 25, 2020, from. https://www.bbc.com/news/uk-52053914

Heymann, D. L., & Shindo, N. (2020). COVID-19: What is next for public health? *The Lancet, 395* (10224), 542–545. https://doi.org/10.1016/S0140-6736(20)30374-3

Islam, F. (2020, March 26). Coronavirus: UK government unveils aid for self-employed. BBC News. Retrieved April 25, 2020, from. https://www.bbc.com/news/uk-52053914

Kinner, S. A., Young, J. T., Snow, K., Southalan, L., Lopez-Acuña, D., Ferreira-Borges, C., & O'Moore, É. (2020). Prisons and custodial settings are part of a comprehensive response to COVID-19. *The Lancet Public Health, 5*(4), e188–e189. https://doi.org/10.1016/S2468-2667(20)30058-X

Rein, L. (2020, April 15). In unprecedented move, Treasury orders Trump's name printed on stimulus check. *Washington Post*. (Retrieved April 26, 2020, from. https://www.washingtonpost.com/politics/coming-to-your-1200-relief-check-donald-j-trumps-name/2020/04/14/071016c2-7e82-11ea-8013-1b6da0e4a2b7_story.html

Animal (Non-human) Companionship for Adults Aging in Place during COVID-19: A Critical Support, a Source of Concern and Potential for Social Work Responses

Dear Editor,

Older adults living in the community are at disproportionate risk for loneliness and isolation and associated increased health risks (Malcolm et al., 2019); this risk has been further exacerbated by the self-isolation recommended during this pandemic (Armitage & Nellums, 2020). However, many older adults living in the community have a potential intervention for such embedded in their lives – their pets. To explore such, the Gerontological Society of America (GSA) convened an international work group of experts in the fields of aging and human–animal interaction beginning in 2016 to develop a roadmap for understanding how pets may positively impact loneliness, social isolation, depression and mobility among older adults (Resnick & McCune, 2019). The National Institute of Aging released an infographic that included pet adoption as a strategy to reduce loneliness and social isolation in older adults (https://www.nia.nih. gov/sites/default/files/social-isolation-infographic-508.pdf). Nationally, pets live in more than half of our homes (American Veterinary Medical Association, 2017–2018). In a study of users of food pantries in Western Pennsylvania 53% of those aged 75 and older were living with one or more pets (Rauktis & Lee, 2019). While pets may be an invaluable source of support for older adults who are experiencing increased isolation and loneliness, unfortunately, most social workers are not trained to include human–animal relationships in assessments and interventions. Social work inclusion of human–animal interaction considerations within the routine practice is increasing, but it is still the exception rather than the rule. In this letter, we present a case for why and how social workers who work with older adults should assess and respond to human–pet interaction; while important on a routine basis, given the current pandemic situation and subsequent increases in isolation experienced by older adults, it is especially crucial to be responsive to their relationships with pets as potential strengths, stressors or both.

A major risk factor, other than COVID infection for older adults living in the community during this pandemic is social isolation (Armitage & Nellums, 2020). Research has consistently shown that social isolation and loneliness in older adults are associated with deleterious physical and mental health outcomes including cardiovascular disease (Thurston, 2009; Udell et al., 2012), depression (Cacioppo et al., 2006) and is a risk factor for accelerated mortality (Pennix et al., 1997). Pets have the potential to be particularly therapeutic for older adults because their pet is a primary source of social, emotional and psychological support (Krause-Parello, 2008; McNicholas, 2014; Rauktis & Lee, 2019). However, not all older adults realize the full benefits that having a pet can provide. Social workers are experts at mobilizing strengths and resources within the social and emotional contexts of clients, and there are numerous ways that they can help leverage and augment the benefits that older adults can experience through the presence of a pet in their homes. Social workers can do such using telephone screenings, check-ins and telemedicine.

Companion animals need to be part of the psychosocial assessment so that the presence of an animal in the home is in the record and the benefits and challenges are known and incorporated into service plans

Pets can be included in genograms and questions about how the pets connect them to the outside world incorporated in the assessment and in the plan (Hodgson et al., 2015). Rauktis (2019) found that pets were more of a social connector for older adults than younger adults in that pets motivated older adults to converse outside the home with neighbors about their pets. With social distancing, these connections can be maintained in virtual or digital ways. For example, Rauktis (2019) reports that one dog owner would call her shut-in friends with her jack Russell terrier on the line. This was the social highlight for both the dog owner, the shut-in and the dog!

Companion animals can be part of goal-directed wellness plans

Dogs need to be walked, cats need active play – walking and bending and tossing are physical activities that can be practiced in the home routinely and in the case of walking outside, in the short distance around the home with protective personal equipment.

Pets are a window into engagement and should be utilized. Rauktis (2019) reports in her study that when she asked older adults to talk about their pet, the response was uniformly positive and their older respondents became visibly brighter. If an isolated older adult appears unwilling to talk about themselves, it is very likely that they will want to talk about their pet/pets.

Planning for fun

In the time of COVID-19, we need to be creative about fun and social workers can brainstorm fun ideas for activities with pets – themed parties, silly photos, writing stories about the pet.

Social workers should also be cognizant of the challenges of aging in place with a pet during the pandemic

Limited or lack of access to pet food may result in feeding their pet human food, decreasing their caloric and protein intake, and human food is not formulated for the nutritional needs of animals. Another challenge is may be reluctant to seek treatment for virus or leave their homes for hospitalization due to concerns about the companion animal.

Ways that social workers can mitigate or prevent some of these challenges are to make connections with the community outreach staff in animal welfare agencies in order to help clients access needed resources such as free pet food and low-cost wellness services for the animals. Having a plan for a trusted person(s) to care for the pet is imperative now. Social workers can help them make a plan as a preventative act instead of waiting for an emergency. The plan would include helping the client create a virtual "go bag" for the pet with food, crate/carrier or leash, toys, authorize power of attorney for care of the pet, vet records and identification and write down pet routines and behaviors.

If the older adult can remain in the home with COVID, they should self-quarantine with the pet then ask a friend or supports to leave food and supplies outside the house and taking dogs for a walk using Protective Precautions. Again, having someone identified to do this before the older adult becomes ill or needs hospitalization is critical as there will not be time to do this when they become acutely ill. Finally, if hospitalization is necessary then the choice is either keep animals in a home with someone coming in and caring for them or moving the pet(s) to another home or boarding. This should be discussed with the older adult prior to a medical crisis as they know their pet best and are not likely to get help or go to the hospital if they feel that their pet will be harmed. We are working on a resource guide at this time for "aging in place with pets in Western Pennsylvania," created by the University of Pittsburgh Hartford Scholar students. Other regions have similar guides and social workers should have this resource at hand during this pandemic.

To summarize, this pandemic has highlighted the import of routinely including the human–animal bond as potentially both a strength and stressor within social work practice with older adults. Through explicitly supporting older adults' relationships with their pets, associated benefits may be leveraged to help ameliorate increases in social isolation, loneliness and other pandemic-related stressors (Hoy-Gerlach et al., 2020). Helping to alleviate stressors experienced by older adults related to having pets can likewise help to preserve having the pet as an ongoing support. In a time when older adults – a population already at disproportionate risk of isolation and associated health issues – are experiencing dramatic increases in isolation due to COVID-19 vulnerability, the inclusion of human–animal bond considerations can be a valuable way to help offset such.

Mary E. Rauktis and Janet Hoy-Gerlach

References

American Veterinary Medical Association (2017-2018). *U.S. pet ownership statistics* https://www.avma.org/resources-tools/reports-statistics/us-pet-ownership-statistics#formulas

Armitage, R., & Nellums, L. B. (2020). COVID-19 and the consequences of isolating the elderly. *The Lancet Public Health*, 5(5), e256. Online first. Published March 19, 2020. https://doi.org/10.1016/S2468-2667(20)30061-X

Cacioppo, J. T., Hughes, M. E., Waite, L. J., Hawkley, L. C., & Thisted, R. A. (2006). Loneliness as a specific risk factor for depressive symptoms: Cross-sectional and longitudinal analyses. *Psychology and Aging*, 21(1), 140–151. https://doi.org/10.1037/0882-7974.21.1.140

Hodgson, K., Barton, L., Darling, M., Antao, V., Kim, F., & Monavvari, A. (2015). Pets' impact on your patients' health: Leveraging benefits and mitigating risk. *Journal of the American Board of Family Medicine*, 28(4), 526–534. https://doi.org/10.3122/jabfm.2015.04.140254

Hoy-Gerlach, J., Rauktis, M. E., & Newhill, C. (2020). (Non-human) Animal companionship: A crucial support for people during the COVID-19 pandemic. *Society Register*, 4(2), 2. Published: Apr 7, 2020. https://doi.org/10.14746/sr.2020.4.2.08

Krause-Parello, C. A. (2008). The mediating effect of pet attachment support between loneliness and general health in older females living in the community. *Journal of Community Health Nursing*, 25(1), 1–14. https://doi.org/10.1080/07370010701836286

Malcolm, M., Frost, H., & Cowie, J. (2019). Loneliness and social isolation causal association with health-related lifestyle risk in older adults: A systematic review and meta-analysis protocol. *Systematic Reviews*, 8(1), 1-8. https://doi.org/10.1186/s13643-019-0968-x

McNicholas, J. (2014). The role of pets in the lives of older people: A review. *Working With Older People*, 18(3), 128–144. https://doi.org/10.1108/WWOP-06-2014-0014

Pennix, B. W., Guralnik, J. M., Ferrucci, L., Simonsick, E. M., Dorly, J. H., Deeg, D., & Wallace, R. B. (1997). Depressive symptoms and physical decline in community-dwelling older persons. *Journal of the American Medical Association, 279*(21), 1720–1726. https://doi.org/10.1001/jama.279.21.1720

Rauktis, M. E., & Lee, H. (2019) *Animal ownership in low-income households: Is here a relationship between human and animal food insecurity?* Project report. University of Pittsburgh School of social work. http://d-scholarship.pitt.edu/35957/

Resnick, B., & McCune, S. (2019). Introduction to the themed issue on human–animal interaction and healthy human aging. *Anthrozoös, 32*(2), 165–168. https://doi.org/10.1080/08927936.2019.156990

Thurston, R. C. (2009). Women, loneliness and Incident coronary heart disease. *Psychosomatic Medicine, 71*(8), 836–842. https://doi.org/10.1097/PSY.0b013e3181b40efc

Udell, J. A., Steg, P. G., Scirica, B., Smith, S. C., Ohman, M., Eagle, K. A., Goto, S., Cho, J. L., Bhattt, D., L. (2012). Living alone and cardiovascular risk in outpatients at risk of or with atherothrombosis. *Archives of Internal Medicine, 172*(14), 1086–1096. https://doi.org/10.1001/archinternmed.2012.2782

Detroit's Efforts to Meet the Needs of Seniors: Macro Responses to a Crisis

Dear Editor,

Social isolation of the poor is endemic to most large American cities. The COVID-19 pandemic lockdown exacerbated the situation for an estimated 3,400 extremely low-income seniors living in high rise apartments in midtown and downtown Detroit, Michigan. Some of the building managers left without notice, others left with insufficient safety instructions. Many of these residents were left to follow the state's shelter-in-place order with only broadcast news to keep them informed and educated about a situation for which they were most vulnerable.

The Senior Housing Preservation – Detroit Coalition (SHP-D), a volunteer organization without paid staff, organized to protect low-income senior housing in the urban core and promote development of naturally occurring affordable housing. But as the COVID-19 pandemic took hold in the city, the coalition found itself asking who should look after the seniors in these buildings. They were left with insufficient personal protection equipment, and an uncertain source of food, medications, and essential hygiene productions; even more important, they lacked companionship at time of high anxiety.

SHP-D issued a statement of concern to alert the City of Detroit, advocates for older adults, and funders that the social isolation of this population could result in death and misery for those locked in their apartments. We called for a well-planned and coordinated response that we believed to be vital to the survival of Detroit's low-income senior population – a sustained effort that needed to last until a vaccine or effective treatment is discovered.

SHP-D has developed a constructive engagement with the City of Detroit in its ongoing efforts to develop new and preserve existing quality, affordable housing for this population. Further, city and state partners have been responsive to SHP-D member concerns about the immediate needs of senior residents as the entire Detroit community addressed the current threat of COVID-19 and the needed stay-at-home strategies. Many in this senior population are often considered Extremely Low-Income (ELI) with annual incomes often under 10,000 USD. Many of these seniors experience chronic health conditions and disparities reflecting a lifetime of poor physical and mental health care. As part of our focus on preserving housing for low-income seniors, SHP-D works to demonstrate the link between stable housing and the health and well-being of seniors, emphasizing the contributions of older adults to the community. The

COVID-19 pandemic environment is a critical example of how health and housing merge.

The City of Detroit responded to our appeal, providing protective masks and COVID-19 testing in the buildings. We have alerted emergency food sources, distributing "quarantine boxes" of food and prepared personal hygiene kits. Wayne State University volunteers initiated a wellness call service to determine the needs and provide another source of contact for seniors.

We issued the following recommendations for long-term support of this vulnerable senior population:

- Identify buildings/populations at greatest risk in terms of lack of resources and building/personnel infrastructure for meeting the challenges of COVID-19 transmission.
- Ensure safety and health of seniors living in low-income residences, including use of common building areas like hallways, elevators, laundry rooms, and mailrooms.
- Develop ways to provide food and essential supplies, allowing residents to remain safe in their homes.
- Leverage ways to reduce social isolation through telecommunications, activities, and other means.
- Recognize the challenge of managing senior housing buildings during the pandemic, and how the illness of frontline staff will affect the safety of residents.
- •Create a communication system to inform seniors about recommended precautions and how to get essential needs met, with the understanding that the population has limited access to online resources.
- Designate a point-of-contact for seniors through a city department or established service provider.
- Mobilize the support of elected officials, philanthropic leaders, and others to help create a sustained emergency safety net for this vulnerable population.

As interdisciplinary professionals working for the health and well-being of older adults in our communities, we continue to advocate for practices and policies that promote the physical and mental health of older Detroiters. Our coalition, founded in 2013, already had experience working together, so mobilizing during the pandemic by increasing meetings, information sharing, and problem solving was welcomed by our active members. Social workers with training in gerontology have great opportunity to participate in coalitions like SHP-D as ways to use their backgrounds and training to be part of concrete solutions.

Thank you for the opportunity to highlight the concerns in Detroit.

Sincerely,

Dennis Archambault

Claudia Sanford

Tam Perry

http://orcid.org/0000-0002-8447-6115

Foregrounding Context in the COVID-19 Pandemic: Learning from Older Adults in Puerto Rico

Dear Editor,

Person-environment fit is a basic principle in both social work practice and the ecological model of human aging. Yet we often privilege the individual over collective, functional over structural, and proximal over distal. This orientation can distract us from important contexts. Herein we describe how older adults' reporting, even and perhaps especially in a semi-structured survey, can serve as a potent corrective. We then offer suggestions for research and practice with this population in the COVID-19 pandemic.

In September 2019, we initiated a study in Puerto Rico to assess the mental health status and needs of community-dwelling older adults two years after Hurricane María. Informed by interviews with community leaders, academics, NGO's, clergy and government officials there, we conducted semi-structured interviews with 154 adults aged 60+ and in-depth narrative interviews with a subsample of 8. Between one-third and one-half of interviewees scored above the cutoffs thresholds for common mental disorders (depression, anxiety, traumatic stress), PTSD and social disconnectedness (loneliness, social isolation, sense of community).

We are preparing to pilot an evidence-based intervention to improve older adults' mental health by strengthening their social connectedness. In reviewing team debriefings, study logs and detailed annotations on the survey instruments, we realized how effortlessly and effectively participants had negotiated our interviews to contextualize their responses. We summarize this context, without which, as Bateson (1988) reminds us, "words and actions have no meaning at all" (p. 15).

On the heels of Hurricane Irma, María struck Puerto Rico with deadly force on September 20, 2017. The island's economy had been in recession for nearly a decade, forcing it into bankruptcy early that year.[1] The poverty rate was 44.4% and older adults were 7 times more likely than younger adults to be poor. Subsequent mass migration of young adults to the mainland had led to 10% population decline, 20% labor force reduction and accelerated population aging (20.7% were 65+ in 2019). Some 4,645 people, mostly older adults and the poor, died in Mariá and its aftermath. Suicides rose 29%–more than doubling for persons aged 65–69 and tripling for those aged 75–79. In the past two years, 51% of all suicides have been for older adults.

---

[1] On the colonial history of Puerto Rico and its relationship with the U.S., see, for example, Cheatham, 2020a; Malaret (1997) and Soto-Crespo (2009).

In July, 2019, the governor was ousted for corruption and scandal. In December and into 2020, the island was wracked by major earthquakes. On March 13, the first case of COVID-19 was confirmed. Despite swift action, by early May unemployment had quadrupled to 37% and the economic toll was estimated at 10 USDB – about 10% of the GDP (Cheatham, 2020b . On June 28, there were 7,066 confirmed cases (221 per capita) (CDC, 2020a). Only 8 states and territories have lower rates, but the gravity of the threat in Puerto Rico lies principally in the aforementioned contexts, which have decimated healthcare infrastructure and contributed to excess disease burden for older adults. As of June 22, 26.5% of confirmed cases were aged 65+, 33.1% were aged 60+ and 53.1% were aged 50+ (Instituto de Estadísticas de Puerto Rico, 2020).

It is unclear why older adults are at higher risk of serious disease and death from COVID-19 (CDC, 2020b ; Promislow, 2020). Sands et al. (2020) discuss three possibile contributors: higher age-related multi-morbidity rates and declines in immune functioning and increased inflammatory pathways; nursing home residency; and health disparities – hospital and mortality rates are two times higher for African Americans and Latinos than non-Latino Whites in the U.S. (Laurencin & McClinton, 2020; see COVID-19 Racial Data Tracker https://covidtracking.com/race).

As fewer Black and Latino older adults live in nursing homes, their higher rates are likely related to current and cumulative disadvantages. Gerontologists have a scientific lexicon for the processes and outcomes of stress, e.g., environmental press, weathering, allostatic load and depletion. Lay accounts are shaped more by individual and collective narratives, at times expressed as culture-specific "idioms of distress." These accounts emanate from an intrinsic human need to find logic and meaning in one's experiences and to have others ratify, share, and even act on their stories.

However unintentionally, our project served as an impromptu, semi-public arena for older adults to accomplish this task.[2] Metonymically standing in and standing up for others like them, they offered *testimonios* to clarify, verify and amplify what Farmer (1996) describes as "the mechanisms through which large-scale social forces crystallize into the sharp, hard surfaces of individual suffering" (p. 263). One central theme was abandonment – by the U.S., their own government, communities, families, and for some, God. As we recontact these older adults to explore the impact of COVID-19, we are acutely aware of how the pandemic can worsen a sense of abandonment, loss and isolation (Hwang et al., 2020). Herewith are several suggestions from our experience for COVID-19 related research and practice with older adults in similar contexts:

---

[2]Fraser and Honneth (2003) offer a useful theoretical approach to this phenomenon.

- Recognize the need to be recognized
- Assess and address mental health problems
- Attend to cues of active *and* passive suicidal ideation
- Recognize personal *and* social grief and suffering
- Encourage reflection on past and current situations
- Include persons with disabilities, including cognitive impairments
- Address added demands and reduced supports among caregivers
- Ask what it means to older adults to be in a 'vulnerable' population and how it affects their decisions about health and safety behaviors.
- Consider the effects of public safety behaviors, e.g., protective face coverings on communication and social distancing on loneliness and isolation.
- Treat context as integral, not only the background of COVID-19.
- Determine how relationships with the state and various civil society sectors affect care quality and preferences, e.g., active treatment, palliative, end-of-life.
- Challenge public rhetoric about the pandemic. To what extent are we really "all in this together?" How 'socially indiscriminate' is COVID19?
- What role do ageism, racism and other interpersonal and inter-group dynamics play for older adults in the unfolding pandemic?

Denise Burnette, Tommy D. Buckley, Humberto E. Fabelo and Mauricio
P. Yabar

References

Bateson, G. (1988). *Mind and nature*. Bantam Books.

Centers for Disease Control and Prevention (CDC). 2020b). *Coronavirus disease 2019 (COVID-19). Groups at higher risk of severe illness*. Retrieved June 17, 2020, from https://www.cdc.gov/coronavirus/2019-ncov/need-extra-precautions/groups-at-higher-risk.html

Centers for Disease Control and Prevention (CDC), 2020a). *United States COVID-19 cases and deaths by state*. Retrived June 27, 2020, from https://www.cdc.gov/covid-data-tracker/index.html#cases

Cheatham, A. (2020b). *The coronavirus challenge for Puerto Rico*. U.S. Council on Foreign Relations. May 12. https://www.cfr.org/in-brief/coronavirus-challenge-puerto-rico 1/5

Cheatham, A. (2020a). *Puerto Rico: A U.S. territory in crisis*. U.S. Council on Foreign Relations. https://www.cfr.org/backgrounder/puerto-rico-us-territory-crisis

Farmer, P. (1996). On suffering and structural violence: A view from below. *Daedalus, 125*(1), (Social suffering (Winter, 1996)), 261–283. MIT Press on behalf of American Academy of Arts & Sciences. Available from: https://www.jstor.org/stable/20027362

Fraser, N., & Honneth, A. (2003). *Redistribution or recognition?: A political-philosophical exchange*. Verso.

Hwang, T.-J., Rabheru, K., Peisah, C., Reichman, W., & Ideda, M. (2020). Loneliness and social isolation during the COVID-19 pandemic. *International Psychogeriatrics, 1-4.* https://doi.org/10.1017/S1041610220000988

Instituto de Estadísticas de Puerto Rico. (2020). *Plataforma de Indicadores COVID-19.* Basado en datos oficiales provistos por el Departamento de Salud de Puerto Rico. Disponible en: https://estadisticas.pr/en/covid-19.

Laurencin, C., & McClinton, A. (2020). The COVID-19 pandemic: A call to action to identify and address racial and ethnic disparities [published online April 18, 2020]. *Journal of Racial and Ethnic Health Disparities, 7*(3), 398–402. https://doi.org/10.1007/s40615-020-00756-0

Malaret, D. (1997). *Theoretical and conceptual lacunae in sociological theories of development: The Puerto Rican anomaly* [Unpublished doctoral dissertation]. Western Michigan University.

Promislow, D. (2020). A geroscience perspective on COVID-19 mortality [published online April 17, 2020]. *The Journals of Gerontology: Series A*, 1-4. https://doi.org/10.1093/gerona/glaa094

Sands, L. P., Albert, S. M., & Suitor, J. J. (2020). Understanding and addressing older adults' needs during COVID-19. *Innovation in Aging, 4*(3), 1–3. Advance Access publication, June 2. https://doi.org/10.1093/geroni/igaa019

Soto-Crespo, R. E. (2009). *Mainland passage: The cultural anomaly of Puerto Rico.* University of Minnesota Press.

An Innovative Telephone Outreach Program to Seniors in Detroit, a City Facing Dire Consequences of COVID-19

Dear Editor,

We write this letter to call attention to the implications of loneliness and social isolation to the wellbeing of minority older adults, especially during the time of Covid-19, and describe our program aimed at mitigating these challenges. Although loneliness is an important emotion to think about at any age, countless studies have shown the detrimental effects loneliness and social isolation can have on older adult's physical and mental health, and even shorten their lifespan (AARP Foundation, n.d.; Cudjoe, 2020; Hawkley & Cacioppo, 2010). Loneliness is a perceived emotion; thus, someone with an active social life filled with events and surrounded by friends can still feel very lonely (Hawkley & Cacioppo, 2010). Therefore, it is particularly important to focus on older adult's perception of loneliness that involves asking about how connected they feel to friends and family, how many individuals do they feel they can talk to, that they can rely on, go to for help, and more (Holt-Lunstad et al., 2010). Prior to Covid-19, the number of isolated older adults was significant at 17% (AARP Foundation, n. d.). The physical and social distancing put in place to reduce the spread of Covid-19 has surely increased this number.

Covid-19 disproportionally affects minority older adults, particularly African Americans, in grave ways. In Detroit, 66% of confirmed Covid-19 cases are among African Americans, and 57% of all cases are Detroiters aged 70 and older. Furthermore, 82% of all deaths within Detroit due to Covid-19 are African American (Detroit Health Department, 2020).

Although advances in technology can help keep us connected, the National Digital Inclusion Alliance (2018) utilized data from the US Census to reveal that almost 30% of households in Detroit do not have any type of broadband internet. Furthermore, at least one in five Detroit households lack broadband subscriptions of any type (including cellular data plans) and currently ranks as the 19th worst connected city in the US.

So how can we help a population that has potential detrimental effects from feelings of loneliness and social isolation, experiencing high disproportional death rates from Covid-19, and has generally limited access to newer technology that could bridge the gap of physical distancing? We would like to share our telephone outreach project that aims to address this very question in hopes that other groups working with older adults can replicate these strategies.

The Healthier Black Elders Center (HBEC) is an NIH funded program located in Detroit, Michigan. Over 20 years ago, the NIH put forth a call for action to increase the participation of minorities in research and the amount of minority scientists conducting research on minority populations. This created various centers across the country that focuses on a particular population. In Michigan, it created the Michigan Center for Urban African American Aging Research (MCUAAAR) that is jointly coordinated by three universities. The Healthier Black Elders Center is the community core of MCUAAAR. HBEC aims to address and reduce health disparities through research and education. We invite older African American adults to join and become members of our program. Typically, we host in-person community events to provide free education for our members, and the larger Detroit older population, on various age-related health topics. Due to Covid-19, we have canceled all in-person events, which has negatively impacted our members because these events provide opportunities for social gathering and strong engagement among older Detroiters. To remain connected and engaged with all 1,300 members of our program, we developed a telephone survey to gain an understanding of how they are experiencing the pandemic to capture both challenges and successes.

We established a team of callers that are making the telephone calls to our HBEC members. The callers consist of university research assistants, students, staff, and older adult community advisory board members. They all received an orientation and training to conduct the telephone survey, collect and submit the data, and connect HBEC members to needed resources. In our survey, we start with open-ended questions such as how they are doing, what unmet needs they may have, what is helping them cope during this time, what has given them strength, and how much of a change has this been. We then use the established short form UCLA loneliness scale and the Lubben social network scale to have quantifiable measures of loneliness and social isolation (Lubben, 1988; Russell, 1996).

Some of our quantitative findings thus far have revealed a majority of HBEC members rate the current situation of Covid-19 as being somewhat stressful (n=124), only sometimes feel that there are people who really understand them (n=131), yet never feel isolated from others (n=149). We also added a question about mask-wearing after starting the outreach program. We have found that **100%** of those contacted since May 28, 2020, report wearing a mask when going out (n=86). Qualitative results will require a more in-depth analysis.

There are a few critical points to this project that are deeply important to everyone involved; it is imperative that we connect with our members to 'check-in' and let them know we are thinking about them during this time, and it is equally important that we are capturing both positive and negative experiences of the pandemic in their own voices. Using a strengths-based perspective, we want to report the challenges and needs, but also the coping strategies and resiliency of older adults during Covid-19. Lastly, and what has turned to be most crucial, we provide our members with relevant resources to address any unmet needs they may have. Many older adults are fearful to leave their homes, and many do not have the means to search online for resources. We have addressed unmet needs by connecting older adults to various community resources such as counseling and therapy services, assistance with completing their taxes, getting their water turned back on, and supplying them with face masks. Most of these connections were simply providing the older adult with the phone number to the relevant organization.

This collective effort has resulted in a deeply rewarding outcome for both the project staff and older adult members. This has provided some students and staff the opportunity to engage with older adults for the first time, which resulted in an enriching learning experience. Our HBEC members have expressed their deep appreciation for the telephone call, many stating that one phone call positively affected their day, week, and even month. Not every call has been easy, as many report talking about grief and loss concerns as Detroit has lost 1,441 residents to date (Detroit Health Department, 2020). Few in the city have not experienced at least one loss or sickness due to Covid-19.

This project has provided the opportunity for innovation in programming to meet the needs of older adults. As many social workers across the world are faced with tailoring their work, we are working with existing resources, a telephone, and volunteers and staff willing to spend time to make these calls. We have heard that these calls are proving to be enriching for both the call recipient and the caller, thus showing a well-known aspect in social work of the importance of relationships and rapport building in practice. This outreach program also makes sure that the voices of older Detroiters are not lost even at the time when stay-at-home orders and restricted movement are part of our context. We would be remiss to overlook the many examples of productive aging evidenced in this outreach program including over half of our callers are older adults (55+), and in the numerous phone calls, we hear of older adults in the community caring for others, making and then donating facemasks, and friendships being formed between caller and call recipient. Thus, our program demonstrates the possibility of coming together as a community in struggling times.

Sincerely,

Vanessa Rorai

ⓘ http://orcid.org/0000-0001-7778-0824

Tam E. Perry

ⓘ http://orcid.org/0000-0002-8447-6115

Funding

This study was supported by a grant from the National Institutes of Health, P30 AG015281, and the Michigan Center for Urban African American Aging Research.

References

AARP Foundation. (n.d.). *Social isolation is more than feeling lonely.* Connect 2 affect. Retrieved June 16, 2020, from https://connect2affect.org

Cudjoe, T. K. M., Roth, D. L., Szanton, S. L., Wolff, J. L., Boyd, C. M., & Thorpe, R. J. (2020). The epidemiology of social isolation: National health and aging trends study. *The Journals of Gerontology: Series B, 75*(1), 107–113. https://doi.org/10.1093/geronb/gby037

Detroit Health Department. (2020). *COVID-19 Dashboard* [Data set]. https://codtableau. detroitmi.gov/t/DHD/views/CityofDetroit-PublicCOVIDDashboard/DemographicCases Dashboard?%3AisGuestRedirectFromVizportal=y&%3Aembed=y

Hawkley, L. C., & Cacioppo, J. T. (2010). Loneliness matters: A theoretical and empirical review of consequences and mechanisms. *Annals of Behavioral Medicine, 40*(2), 218 227. https:// doi.org/10.1007/s12160-010-9210-8

Holt-Lunstad, J., Smith, T. B., & Layton, J. B. (2010). Social relationships and mortality risk: A meta-analytic review. *PLoS Medicine, 7*(7), e1000316. https://doi.org/10.1371/journal.pmed. 1000316

Lubben, J. E. (1988). Assessing social networks among elderly populations. *Family & Community Health, 11*(3), 42–52. https://doi.org/10.1097/00003727-198811000-00008

National Digital Inclusion Alliance. (2018). *Worst connected cities 2018.* Retrieved June 16, 2020, from https://www.digitalinclusion.org/worst-connected-2018/

Russell, D. W. (1996). UCLA loneliness Scale (Version 3): Reliability, validity, and factor structure. *Journal of Personality Assessment, 66*(1), 20–40. https://doi.org/10.1207/ s15327752jpa6601_2

Healthcare Concerns of Older Adults during the COVID-19 Outbreak in Low- and Middle-Income Countries: Lessons for Health Policy and Social Work

Francis Arthur-Holmes ⓘ, Michael Kwesi Asare Akaadom, Williams Agyemang-Duah ⓘ, Kwaku Abrefa Busia ⓘ, and Prince Peprah ⓘ

ABSTRACT

Older people have been identified to be one of the most vulnerable population groups to the 2019 novel coronavirus (COVID-19). At the same time, more health workers in low-and middle-income countries (LMICs) including Ghana are contracting COVID-19. This poses healthcare utilization concerns for older adults. As a result, many older adults are changing their health-seeking behavior by staying at home and resorting to informal healthcare such as the use of traditional therapies and over-the-counter medicines for self-treatment or to boost their immune system. This commentary calls for social workers to collaborate with health authorities and community pharmacists to develop social and health programs to increase older adults' access to healthcare during the COVID-19 crisis. Policies are also required to deal with the pandemic and its impact on health systems in LMICs for both short and long term. We have suggested in this commentary how governments, health institutions, and local authorities in LMICs can address the healthcare concerns of older adults during this and any future pandemic.

Introduction

In low- and middle-income countries (LMICs), the capacity of health systems to deliver effective healthcare services is a challenge. The emergence of the 2019 Coronavirus disease (COVID-19) has exposed the healthcare capacities and also seems to aggravate the existing challenges in the health sectors and systems in these countries. This is because there has been additional burden on primary health systems resulting in the diversion of health services (resources) toward emergency response to the COVID-19 pandemic. Undoubtedly, this will freeze the already limited access to healthcare. The COVID-19 pandemic, as United Nations Development Program (UNDP) (2020) reports, is "more than a global health emergency" and has, therefore, brought the world to a level where all humans are required to adhere to the preventive measures. These include regular washing of hands with soap, using alcohol-based hand sanitizers, wearing of face masks, and engaging in healthy lifestyle (such as eating healthy food, consuming more fruits and vegetables and exercising regularly to boost the immune system).

Reports from the World Health Organization (WHO) and empirical evidence have variously shown that COVID-19 as a life-threatening respiratory illness has huge health and social impacts on older adults who generally have poorer health outcomes and weak immune systems that make them prone to infections (Armitage & Nellums, 2020; Arthur-Holmes & Agyemang-Duah, 2020). This suggests that it is critical to protect older adults during the pandemic and thus, healthcare systems need to be strengthened with facilities and trained health personnel to mitigate the spread of the virus. Despite the growing studies and commentaries on COVID-19, perspectives on healthcare concerns of older adults during the COVID-19 outbreak in developing countries remain nascent and are undocumented. Drawing on COVID-19 situations and health challenges in Ghana and other LMICs, we provide commentary on how older adults' fear of getting exposed to COVID-19 influence their health-seeking behavior and then address their healthcare concerns.

Healthcare concerns and health-seeking behavior of older adults during the Covid-19 pandemic

Older people are faced with both non-communicable and communicable diseases. These diseases and other health problems include cognitive impairment, hypertension, diabetes, anemia, chronic respiratory diseases, cancers, ischemic heart diseases, and kidney problems (Aboderin & Beard, 2015). During this pandemic, older people, especially those who have chronic non-communicable diseases will still require regular care and special attention from their health professionals and informal caregivers to improve their health or manage their illness. However, the outbreak of COVID-19 has infused fear into older people, particularly through the evidence and reports that they have higher fatality rates should they get infected with the virus.

The spread of the disease outstrips the healthcare capacity of most LMICs, particularly those in sub-Saharan Africa to treat it and subsequently causes a shift in attention from normal patients to COVID-19 patients. For instance, in Nigeria, the state hospitals are poorly invested and managed with inadequate equipment and as a result, private hospitals are involved in treating COVID-19 patients. However, the health personnel who treat COVID-19 patients in the private health facilities lack adequate facilities and required training to treat infectious diseases. That has exposed healthcare workers to the virus and thus they have become the source of diffusion of the virus to their families (Ifijeh et al., 2020). As of 30 April 2020, 113 health workers in Nigeria had been infected with the virus (Abu-bashal, 2020). In South Africa, over 500 health workers have contracted the virus as of 06 May 2020 (Isilow, 2020). Also, in India, 90 health professionals have been infected with the virus as of 12 April 2020 (Bhasin, 2020). It could be argued that lack of health resources and improper supply of personal protective equipment to health workers in these countries are responsible for the spread of the virus to health workers.

The situation concerning Ghana's healthcare system is not different from these LMICs which have poor healthcare systems. As of 18 July 2020, over 2,000 health workers in Ghana had been infected with COVID-19 (Adamu, 2020). Because frontline health workers were getting infected with the virus, some public health facilities, particularly those in Accra and Kumasi were closed for some days and opened after disinfection exercises. However, the poor healthcare system in Ghana and other LMICs have caused older adults to have mistrust in the delivery of formal healthcare services. This situation coupled with the challenges of accessing healthcare facilities (such as long distance to access healthcare, long waiting hours, poor attitude of health workers and transportation cost) (Agyemang-Duah et al., 2019) and the fear of exposure to the virus at public healthcare facilities are causing many older adults to stay at home and find the best possible alternative treatment for their illnesses.

It is important to note that after the Government of Ghana lifted the 3-week partial lockdown on 13 April 2020, the cases of COVID −19 have increased from 636 to 27,060 cases with 145 deaths as of 19 July 2020. Older adults are now more scared of the virus than before as some of them have expressed their worry on Radio Stations that they live in a period of each one for him/herself, where the financial capacity of the country matters more to the government than her citizens. As Gyasi (2020, p. 1) emphasizes, "the exponential rate of COVID-19 cases and deaths in Ghana have engendered intense fear and anxiety among the at-risk populations with serious implications for mental health and well-being of older people." In light of this, many older adults are compelled to purchase orthodox medicine at pharmacies to "treat self-recognized or self-diagnosed conditions or symptoms" (Ruiz, 2010, p. 315). As is the case of the COVID-19 pandemic, older adults may tend to self-medicate based on advice and recommendation from their social support networks such as family members, friends, and neighbors. Arthur-Holmes and Agyemang-Duah (2020) argue that social networks play a critical role in providing welfare services, healthcare decisions, and physical movement supports to older adults as they [older adults] would need to depend on their social relations to improve their welfare and health conditions during the pandemic.

Those who have fears of getting infected with the virus at the public health facilities may opt for various modalities of health treatment at a private health facility though at a high cost. Many older adults are also increasing their use of traditional medicine as a means of boosting their immune system and managing their ailments. Traditional medicine is usually bought at herbal shops or markets and sometimes prepared at home (Gyasi et al., 2011). In Africa, Madagascar has been able to develop a herbal medicine, called COVID-Organics drink, to fight against the COVID-19 pandemic. However, the efficacy and safety of the drug remain a subject of national and international discussions and debates especially among the scientific community. In Ghana, for example, steps have been taken to develop local herbal medicines to boost the immune system of COVID-19 patients and the general population. As Gyasi et al. (2011) and Peprah et al. (2019) assert, people consume traditional medicine because of its perceived less adverse side effects, availability, neutrality, and efficacy. Yet, it is crucial for health institutions, the Traditional Medicine Practice Council (TPMC) and other relevant stakeholders to advise older adults about the efficacy and safety of herbal medicine in curing COVID-19 or boosting their immune system. The consumption of herbal medicines or mixtures which have not undergone scientific experiment and approval processes must be discouraged.

Addressing the healthcare concerns of older adults during the COVID-19 pandemic

Health institutions, social welfare departments and governments in LMICs may need to develop health and social intervention programs that will increase older adults' use of public healthcare facilities and also eliminate their fears of getting infected with the virus from health workers. We recommend that in communities where there are no hospitals or clinics for older adults to access formal healthcare, the government and local authorities should build health posts or community-based health planning and service (CHPS) compounds for those communities to enable older adults who may feel reluctant to travel to access formal healthcare at public hospitals or clinics in other communities. Considering this suggestion, governments and health institutions in LMICs must provide these facilities with trained health professionals and organize COVID-19 programs on various media outlets in communities to encourage older adults to obtain healthcare at health posts or CHPS compounds.

State leaders in LMICs may need to build more health facilities to deal with thisand any future pandemic. In Ghana, for instance, the government has decided to complete abandoned health facilities – hospitals and clinics – and build new ones. In all, 111 new health facilities are to be completed to improve the health capacity of the country. It is important that state leaders in other LMICs improve their public health policies and ensure that existing health facilities are adequately resourced in order to meet the increasing demands of patient care.

Moreover, there is the need to increase the COVID-19 testing centers preferably at every district and regional hospitals in LMICs for early detection and treatment. Pharmaceutical laws against over-the-counter drug purchases must be enforced during and after this pandemic to reduce self-medication habits. That notwithstanding, community pharmacists together with local authorities must encourage older adults to consult pharmacists about the medicines they tend to self-medicate with for their own safety during the pandemic. Since self-medication practices may increase in this period, community pharmacists and TMPC may also need to engage in health sensitization programs to advise older adults about the use of traditional medicine to cure illnesses and improve the immune system unless it is approved by relevant authority, like the Food and Drugs Authority or Institutions in LMICs.

Given that the increasing mobile phones and internet penetration in both urban and rural areas and the prospects of mobile health application in LMICs, health decision-makers should endeavor to explore and develop tele-medicine tools such as mhealth and ehealth to open access to healthcare in the pandemic and post-pandemic era.

Furthermore, governments in various LMICs must collaborate with various media outlets to increase public awareness of the COVID-19 outbreak and ensure that the right information about the disease and older adults is disseminated. In view of this, local authorities and social workers can play a crucial role in educating older adults with proper information on the disease and the need to access formal healthcare to improve their health. There is also the need for social workers and social protection agencies to extend their welfare services by collaborating with health professionals and local authorities to provide psychological and emotional support to older adults who may be having psychological and mental problems during this pandemic.

Conclusion

Given the fact that older adults are vulnerable to infectious diseases, the COVID-19 pandemic has posed health concerns for older adults in LMICs. As is the case of any pandemic, this pandemic is changing older adults' health-seeking behavior. As such, many older adults may likely resort to informal healthcare through self-medication or consultation of traditional medicine practitioners for treatment to avoid contracting the virus from health workers. Older adults should, therefore, be encouraged through COVID-19 sensitization programs to visit CHPS compounds or health posts in their communities if they feel reluctant to visit public hospitals for treatment with the fear of getting infected with the virus at various health facilities. Governments in LMICs must use the COVID-19 crisis as an avenue to improve their public health policies, strengthen their healthcare systems and develop social and health intervention programs to enhance the welfare of older adults.

Disclosure statement

The authors declare no conflicts of interest.

ORCID

Francis Arthur-Holmes ⓘ http://orcid.org/0000-0002-5099-4555
Williams Agyemang-Duah ⓘ http://orcid.org/0000-0001-8658-004X
Kwaku Abrefa Busia ⓘ http://orcid.org/0000-0003-2667-7338
Prince Peprah ⓘ http://orcid.org/0000-0002-3816-2713

References

Aboderin, A. G., & Beard, J. (2015). Older people's health in sub-Saharan Africa. *The Lancet*, *385*(9968), e9–e11. https://doi.org/10.1016/S0140-6736(14)61602-0

Abu-bashal, A. (2020).*Nigeria: 113 healthcare workers infected with COVID-19*. Anadolu Agency. https://www.aa.com.tr/en/africa/nigeria-113-healthcare-workers-infected-with-covid-19/1825398#

Adamu, Z. (2020). Over 2,000 healthcare workers in Ghana have been infected with coronavirus. C.N.N News 18 July. https://edition.cnn.com/2020/07/18/africa/ghana-healthcare-workers-coronavirus/index.html

Agyemang-Duah, W., Mensah, C. M., Peprah, P., Arthur, F., & Abalo, E. M. (2019). Facilitators of and barriers to the use of healthcare services from a user and provider perspective in Ejisu-Juaben municipality, Ghana. *Journal of Public Health*, *27*(2), 133–142. https://doi.org/10.1007/s10389-018-0946-0

Armitage, R., & Nellums, L. B. (2020). COVID-19 and the consequences of isolating the elderly. *The Lancet Public Health*, *5*(5), e256. https://doi.org/10.1016/S2468-2667(20)30061-X

Arthur-Holmes, F., & Agyemang-Duah, W. (2020). Reaching older adults during the COVID-19 pandemic through social networks and Social Security Schemes in Ghana: Lessons for considerations. *Journal of Gerontological Social Work*, 1–3. https://doi.org/10.1080/01634372.2020.1764689

Bhasin, S. (2020). *90 Health Workers Infected With COVID-19, Total Cases Over 8,000 in India*. NDTV. https://www.ndtv.com/india-news/coronavirus-india-coronavirus-cases-in-india-cross-8-000-mark-34-dead-in-24-hours-2210282

Gyasi, R. M. (2020). Fighting COVID-19: Fear and internal conflict among older adults in Ghana. *Journal of Gerontological Social Work*, 1–3. https://doi.org/10.1080/01634372.2020.1766630

Gyasi, R. M., Mensah, C. M., Osei-Wusu Adjei, P., & Agyemang, S. (2011). Public perceptions of the role of traditional medicine in the health care delivery system in Ghana. *Global Journal of Health Science*, *3*(2), 40–49.

Ifijeh, M., Ajimotokan, O., & Ezigbo, O. (2020). *Nigeria: Concerns mount over treatment of COVID-19 patients by private hospitals*. THISDAY. https://allafrica.com/stories/202004160662.html

Isilow, H. (2020). *Over 500 South African health workers contract COVID-19*. Anadolu Agency. https://www.aa.com.tr/en/africa/over-500-s-african-health-workers-contract-covid-19/ 1831768

Peprah, P., Agyemang-Duah, W., Arthur-Holmes, F., Budu, H. I., Abalo, E. M., Okwei, R., & Nyonyo, J. (2019). 'We are nothing without herbs': A story of herbal remedies use during pregnancy in rural Ghana. *BMC Complementary and Alternative Medicine*, *19*(1), 1–12. https://doi.org/10.1186/s12906-019-2476-x

Ruiz, M. E. (2010). Risks of self-medication practices. *Current Drug Safety*, *5*(4), 315–323. https://doi.org/10.2174/157488610792245966

United Nations Development Program (UNDP) (2020). *COVID-19: New UNDP data dashboards reveal huge disparities among countries in ability to cope and recover*. UNDP. https://www.undp.org/content/undp/en/home/news-centre/news/2020/COVID19_UNDP_data_dashboards_reveal_disparities_among_countries_to_cope_and_recover.html

Geriatric Health in Bangladesh during COVID-19: Challenges and Recommendations

Md Mahbub Hossain, Hoimonty Mazumder⬤, Samia Tasnim, Tasmiah Nuzhath, and Abida Sultana

ABSTRACT

The novel coronavirus disease (COVID-19) is impacting health globally, whereas older adults are highly susceptible and more likely to have adverse health outcomes. In Bangladesh, the elderly population has been increasing over the past few decades, who often live with poor socioeconomic conditions and inadequate access to healthcare services. These disparities are likely to increase amid COVID-19, which may result in high mortality and morbidity among Bangladeshi older adults. We recommend that multifaceted interventions should be adopted for strengthening social care and health systems approach to ensure wellbeing, promote preventive measures, and facilitate access to healthcare among older adults in Bangladesh. Such multipronged measures would require policy-level commitment and collaborative efforts of health and social care providers and institutions to protect health and wellbeing among this vulnerable population during the COVID-19 pandemic.

The novel coronavirus disease (COVID-19) is a major global health concern, especially for older adults who share a major proportion of mortality and morbidity in this pandemic (World Health Organization, 2020a). COVID-19 imposes unique challenges to low- and middle-income countries (Mazumder, Hossain et al., 2020), leaving Bangladesh with no exception. It is the eighth-most populous country in the world, with more than 162 million population (World Health Organization, 2020b). In 2016, the life expectancy of Bangladeshi males and females became 71 and 74 years, respectively (World Health Organization, 2020b), which is much higher than a national average of 46.5 years in 1971 when the country got independence (The World Bank, 2019). This can be attributable to notable success in terms of reducing child and maternal mortality, infectious diseases, and malnutrition in the past 49 years, which is also known as Bangladesh Paradox (Hossain et al., 2018). However, despite a significant improvement in the overall population health and increased life expectancy, geriatric health problems are still under-recognized in Bangladesh (Barikdar et al., 2016). In this article, we describe unique challenges for Bangladeshi older adults during COVID-19 and discuss potential strategies addressing the same.

In the sociocultural context of Bangladesh, older adults are generally dependent on their family members, which limits the autonomy and abilities for decision-making regarding their own health (Ellickson, 1988). This critically affects their health and quality of living. During COVID-19, socioeconomic challenges like unemployment and poverty are increasing in Bangladesh (The World Bank, 2020), which is impacting the householders as well as older adults living with their families. Moreover, in the absence of an organized and universal social care program, Bangladeshi older adults continue to experience the indirect socioeconomic burden of COVID-19.

Another critical challenge is the high burden of noncommunicable diseases among older adults in Bangladesh (Mazumder, Murshid et al., 2020; Taskin et al., 2014). As the health outcomes of COVID-19 is poorer among people with preexisting conditions (World Health Organization, 2020a), Bangladeshi older adults remain highly vulnerable to adverse health outcomes in this pandemic. Furthermore, as the country is experiencing community transmission of COVID-19 (UN News, 2020), community-dwelling older adults are highly susceptible to the infection and associated mortality.

Lastly, older adults in Bangladesh may lack mobility and access to care amid COVID-19. As the nation has no home-based care program for older adults, seeking institutional services remain the only option for someone who is experiencing any kind of health problems. Moreover, nationwide travel restrictions and limited availability of transportations during this pandemic have made it difficult to access healthcare centers that are located mainly in the urban areas, whereas more than sixty-three percent of the population lives in rural areas of Bangladesh (The World Bank, 2016). In addition, many of the tertiary care centers are transforms into COVID-19 hospitals, where access to regular care services has become limited (Dhaka Tribune, 2020). Therefore, older adults in Bangladesh are less likely to receive timely and appropriate care for COVID-19 and other health problems.

These challenges highlight some of the major challenges that Bangladeshi older adults are experiencing amid COVID-19. Many of those can be explained by evaluating the preexisting health disparities for older people, whereas some of them are aggravating as COVID-19 has impacted socioeconomic conditions and health systems. As more people are approaching to elderhood as well as increased susceptibility to COVID-19, these challenges should be considered for effective policymaking ensuring better health and social care for older adults in Bangladesh. We propose the following recommendations for strengthening geriatric care during COVID-19 in Bangladesh:

(1) Introducing a comprehensive health and social care program for older adults who are dependent on their families or have no sources of income

(2) Strengthening existing social care programs that directly or indirectly support older adults based on the special challenges during COVID-19

(3) Mobilizing community resources like religious institutions and voluntary organizations to improve social care and rapid response to affected or vulnerable older adults during COVID-19

(4) Launching mass media programs like radio shows, television programs, and online events promoting education and awareness on geriatric wellbeing, self-care, and preventive measures for COVID-19

(5) Initiating telemedicine services and remote health consultations for older adults

(6) Educating and empowering informal caregivers to older adults to promote preventive practices and improve access to health services for older adults

(7) Strengthening public health surveillance for COVID-19 among older adults with enhancing diagnostic capacities for this population

(8) Improving collaborations among community health centers and advanced care facilities for effective referral and clinical care

(9) Providing dedicated ambulance services for transporting suspected or diagnosed cases of COVID-19 to the nearest healthcare organization

(10) Prioritizing geriatric care in health and social policymaking for COVID-19 to ensure policy-level resources and support for measures adopted by the community and institutional stakeholders

Geriatric health problems are highly prevalent in Bangladesh, whereas institutional and social capacities to address the same remain limited (Bilkis, 2020; Mazumder, Murshid et al., 2020; Taskin et al., 2014). During the COVID-19 pandemic, these gaps may increase manifolds and result in high mortality and morbidity among older adults who are highly susceptible to infection and less likely to receive adequate care. To maintain the population health gains through preventive measures in the past decades, the policymakers and other key stakeholders must address the geriatric care needs amid the COVID-19 pandemic. Nonetheless, health and social care providers and institutions may play vital roles in policy advocacy and service delivery, promoting geriatric care during COVID-19. Bangladesh has a long history of effective public health measures despite socioeconomic challenges, which should be reinforced in decision-making processes to protect the health of the Bangladeshi older adults in the era of the COVID-19 pandemic.

Funding

No funding was received at any stage of preparing this letter

ORCID

Hoimonty Mazumder ⓘ http://orcid.org/0000-0003-3787-3780

References

Barikdar, A., Ahmed, T., & Lasker, S. P. (2016). The situation of the elderly in Bangladesh. *Bangladesh Journal of Bioethics, 7*(1), 27–36. https://doi.org/10.3329/bioethics.v7i1.29303

Bilkis. (2020). *Lifestyle and depression in urban elderly of selected district of Bangladesh. Mymensingh medical journal: MMJ, 29*(1), 177.Retrieved from https://www.researchgate.net/publication/338514812_Lifestyle_and_Depression_in_Urban_Elderly_of_Selected_District_of_Bangladesh

Dhaka Tribune. (2020). *Kurmitola general hospital soon to treat Covid-19 patients only | Dhaka Tribune.* Retrieved from https://www.dhakatribune.com/bangladesh/dhaka/2020/04/02/kurmitola-general-hospital-soon-to-treat-covid-19-patients-only

Ellickson, J. (1988). Never the twain shall meet: Aging men and women in Bangladesh. *Journal of Cross-Cultural Gerontology, 3*(1), 53–70. https://doi.org/10.1007/BF00116960

Hossain, M. M., Sultana, A., & Munzur-, E.-M. (2018, October 1). Revitalising general practice in Bangladesh: Complementing 'the Bangladesh Paradox. *British Journal of General Practice, 68* (675), 482. Royal College of General Practitioners. https://doi.org/10.3399/bjgp18X699173

Mazumder, H., Hossain, M. M., & Das, A. (2020). Geriatric care during public health emergencies: Lessons learned from novel Corona Virus Disease (COVID-19) pandemic. *Journal of Gerontological Social Work,* 1–2. (Routledge). https://doi.org/10.1080/01634372.2020.1746723.

Mazumder, H., Murshid, M.-E., Faizah, F., & Hossain, M. M. (2020). Geriatric mental health in Bangladesh: A call for action. *International Psychogeriatrics, 32*(5), 1–2. https://doi.org/10.1017/s1041610220000423

Taskin, T., Biswas, T., Siddiquee, A. T., Islam, A., & Alam, D. (2014). *Chronic non-communicable diseases among the elderly in Bangladesh old age homes.* Common Ground Research Networks. Retrieved from https://cgscholar.com/bookstore/works/chronic-noncommunicable-diseases-among-the-elderly-in-bangladesh-old-age-homes

UN News. (2020). *From bustling streets to lockdown: Bangladesh and the UN mobilize to fight COVID-19: A UN resident coordinator blog | | UN News.* Retrieved from https://news.un.org/en/story/2020/04/1062552

The World Bank. (2016). *Rural population (% of total population) Bangladesh.* United Nations. Retrieved from https://data.worldbank.org/indicator/SP.RUR.TOTL.ZS?locations=BD

The World Bank. (2019). *Life expectancy at birth, total (years) - Bangladesh | Data.* World Bank Group. Retrieved from https://data.worldbank.org/indicator/SP.DYN.LE00.IN?locations=BD

The World Bank. (2020). *Bangladesh must ramp up COVID-19 action to protect its people, revive economy.* World Bank Group. Retrieved from https://www.worldbank.org/en/news/press-release/2020/04/12/bangladesh-must-act-now-to-lessen-covid-19-health-impacts

World Health Organization. (2020a). Statement – Older people are at highest risk from COVID-19, but all must act to prevent community spread.

World Health Organization. (2020b). WHO Bangladesh country profile. *WHO.* https://www.who.int/countries/bgd/en/

Lessons for Averting the Delayed and Reduced Patronage of non-COVID-19 Medical Services by Older People in Ghana

Dear Editor,

COVID-19, commonly known as the novel Coronavirus which originated in Wuhan, China in December 2019 has become a severe public health emergency for citizens, societies and the global community at large (Arthur-Holmes & Agyemang-Duah, 2020; Masroor, 2020; Morgan, 2020). The pandemic is imposing a heavy burden on individuals and societies, and putting healthcare systems under severe strain. Governments around the world including that of Ghana are trying to figure out a way to fight this deadly pandemic and what role they can play. While some countries appear to have had some success in slowing the rate of infection, others are far from that. The virus has proved deadliest for older people with some researchers having further theorized that weather conditions could have something to do with the spread while others suggested that population density and the degree of physical contact societies are accustomed to provide fertile grounds for transmission. In effect, populations all over the world are encouraged to stay at home to reduce the spread of the virus and in some cases postpone all nonessential activities (Agyemang-Duah et al., 2020; Morgan, 2020). These measures were strengthened by partial lockdowns in many countries including the then epicenters of the virus in Ghana (Greater Accra, Greater Kumasi Metropolitan Area and its contiguous Districts and Kasoa).

Consequently, the COVID-19 pandemic has dramatically changed how outpatient care is delivered in healthcare practices (Luke Messac et al., 2020). At the onset of the COVID-19 pandemic, it was recommended that healthcare systems prioritize urgent visits and delay elective care to mitigate the spread of COVID-19 in healthcare settings. In jurisdictions where it was possible, they also converted in-person visits to telehealth visits. For their part, many patients are also avoiding visits because they do not want to leave their homes and risk exposure to the deadly virus that has killed nearly 703,374 people globally (Worldometer, 2020). Also influencing both provider and patient behaviour is the evolving local and state recommendations restricting travel and non-essential services. A consequence of the pandemic has been the under-utilization of important medical services for patients with non-COVID -19-related urgent and emergent health needs (Deepthi et al., 2020; De Filippo et al., 2020; Luke Messac et al., 2020).

In Ghana where the pandemic has killed 215 people with over 41,404 infections, there is much apprehension among the majority of the citizens, particularly among older people (Ghana Health Service, 2020). This has translated to reduced healthcare utilization among non-COVID-19 patients. Globally, older people are noted to suffer a wide array of psychological distresses, chronic conditions and multimorbidities (Adeoye, 2015; Banerjee, 2015; McCracken & Phillips, 2017) which possibly increases their demand for healthcare. In Ghana also, this argument has been supported by scholars such as (Agyemang-Duah et al., 2019; Gyasi & Phillips, 2020; Gyasi et al., 2019). With the low level of mHealth (a variant of telehealth) usage in Ghana (Peprah et al., 2020), a sustained decline in healthcare utilization among non-COVID-19 patients could be more disastrous than the COVID-19 pandemic itself. It is therefore imperative for new policies to encourage older people in need of non-COVID-19 care to seek healthcare under supervised conditions to avert another catastrophic scenario especially in the face of the limited operationalization of telehealth services in Ghana. In line with this, the following measures must be taken to promote non-COVID-19 care in the face of the COVID-19 pandemic (particularly among older people).

First, as the pandemic lingers on, healthcare systems in Ghana must balance the need to provide necessary services while minimizing the risk of exposure by patients and healthcare personnel (HCP). With the incidence and effects of COVID-19 varying among communities, healthcare systems in Ghana must consider the local level transmission of COVID-19 when making decisions about the provision of non-COVID-19 medical services. Secondly, care must be provided without delay and, if feasible, services must be shifted to facilities less affected by COVID-19 in instances where deferral of in-person care could highly result in patient harm. In instances where deferral of in-person care has less likelihood of resulting in patient harm, arrangements must be made for in-person care as soon as feasible with priority for at-risk populations (older people). Where applicable, patients should resort to telehealth. Finally, where deferral of in-person care is unlikely to result in patient harm, such medical services must be deferred until community transmission of the virus decreases. The comprehensive implementation of these recommendations holds much promise for reducing non-COVID-19 health complications and deaths consequential of delayed or reduced healthcare utilization, particularly among older people; who have been identified with higher demand for healthcare services.

Sincerely,

Anthony Kwame Morgan

ⓘ http://orcid.org/0000-0001-
7904-9955

Beatrice Aberinpoka Awafo

References

Adeoye, B. D. (2015). Demographic characteristics as determinants of the use of health care services: A case of Nsukka, Southeast Nigeria. *Open Journal of Social Sciences*, *3*(12), 23–28. https://doi.org/10.4236/jss.2015.312003

Agyemang-Duah, W., Morgan, A. K., Oduro, J. A., Peprah, P., & Fordjour, A. A. (2020). Re-integrating older adults who have recovered from the novel coronavirus into society in the context of stigmatization: Lessons for health and social actors in Ghana. *Journal of Gerontological Social Work*, 1–3. https://doi.org/10.1080/01634372.2020.1779163

Agyemang-Duah, W., Peprah, C., & Peprah, P. (2019). Barriers to formal healthcare utilisation among poor older people under the livelihood empowerment against poverty programme in the Atwima Nwabiagya District of Ghana. *BMC Public Health*, *19*(1), 1–12. https://doi.org/10.1186/s12889-019-7437-2

Arthur-Holmes, F., & Agyemang-Duah, W. (2020). Reaching older adults during the COVID-19 pandemic through social networks and social security schemes in Ghana: Lessons for considerations. *Journal of Gerontological Social Work*, 1–3. https://doi.org/10.1080/01634372.2020.1764689

Banerjee, S. (2015). Multimorbidity-older adults need health care that can count past one. *The Lancet*, *385*(9968), 587–589. https://doi.org/10.1016/S0140-6736(14)61596-8

De Filippo, O., D'Ascenzo, F., Angelini, F., Bocchino, P. P., Conrotto, F., Saglietto, A., Campo, G., Gallone, G., Verardi, R., Gaido, L., Iannaccone, M., Galvani, M., Ugo, F., Barbero, U., Infantino, V., Olivotti, L., Mennuni, M., Gili, S., Infusino, F., De Ferrari, G. M., & Secco, G. G. (2020). Reduced rate of hospital admissions for ACS during Covid-19 outbreak in Northern Italy. *New England Journal of Medicine*, *383*(1), 88–89. https://doi.org/10.1056/NEJMc2009166

Deepthi, R., Mendagudli, R. R., Kundapur, R., & Modi, B. (2020). Primary health care and COVID-19 pandemic. *International Journal of Health Systems and Implementation Research*, *4*(1), 20–29. https://ijhsir.ahsas-pgichd.org/index.php/ijhsir/article/view/84/77

Ghana Health Service (2020). *COVID-19 updates in Ghana - Ghana health service*. Retrieved August 12, 2020, from https://ghanahealthservice.org/covid19/

Gyasi, R. M., & Phillips, D. R. (2020). Demography, socioeconomic status and health services utilisation among older Ghanaians: Implications for health policy. *Ageing International*, *45*(1), 50–71. https://doi.org/10.1007/s12126-018-9343-9

Gyasi, R. M., Phillips, D. R., & David, R. (2019). Explaining the gender gap in health services use among Ghanaian community-dwelling older cohorts. *Women & Health*, *59*(10), 1089–1104. https://doi.org/10.1080/03630242.2019.1587666

Luke Messac, M. D., Knopov, A., & Horton, M. (2020). Delayed care-seeking for non-COVID illnesses in Rhode Island. *Rhode Island Medical Journal*, *103*(4), 10–11. http://www.rimed.org/rimedicaljournal/2020/05/2020-05-10-commentary-messac.pdf

Masroor, S. (2020). Collateral damage of COVID-19 pandemic: Delayed medical care. *Journal of Cardiac Surgery*, *35*(6), 1345–1347. https://doi.org/10.1111/jocs.14638

McCracken, K., & Phillips, D. R. (2017). *Global health: An introduction to current and future trends*. Routledge.

Morgan, A. K. (2020). Making COVID-19 prevention etiquette of social distancing a reality for the homeless and slum dwellers in Ghana: Lessons for consideration. *Local Environment*, *25* (7), 536–539. https://doi.org/10.1080/13549839.2020.1789854

Peprah, P., Abalo, E. M., Agyemang-Duah, W., Budu, H. I., Appiah-Brempong, E., Morgan, A. K., & Akwasi, A. G. (2020). Lessening barriers to healthcare in rural Ghana: Providers and users' perspectives on the role of mHealth technology. A qualitative exploration. *BMC Medical Informatics and Decision Making*, *20*(27), 1–12. https://doi.org/10.1186/s12911-020-1040-4

Worldometer. (2020). *Coronavirus death toll and trends – worldometer*. Worldometer. Retrieved August 5, 2020, from https://www.worldometers.info/coronavirus/coronavirus-death-toll/

Index

Acquired Immunodeficiency Syndrome
(AIDS) 81, 116; *see also* Human
Immunodeficiency Virus (HIV)
adult children 11, 43
adult day services 46
adult population 10, 15, 63, 75
advance care planning 18–19
advanced home care 139
African Americans 114, 119, 228–229
ageism 2, 9–11, 21, 26, 57, 110, 119, 142,
188, 201, 226
ageist language 9, 12
AGESW 58, 60; leadership 57
aging 9–12, 25–26, 28, 32, 36–37, 65, 69–71,
74–75, 89, 102–103, 128–129, 141–143,
195, 209–210, 217–219, 224, 229–230;
diversity in 89
Agyemang-Duah, W. 234
Alzheimer's Disease and related dementia
(ADRD) 211–213
American Sign Language (ASL) 105
animal (non-human) companionship 217
Arthur-Holmes, F. 234
assisted living facilities (ALFs) 74–75
Ayalon, L. 26

Bangladesh 239–241; geriatric health
in 239
Bateson, G. 224
bilingual social workers 96
Black, Latinx, and Older Adults of Color
(BLOAC) 92–94
Black adults 192–194
Black populations 111
Brown, L. X. Z. 10

caregivers 17, 20–21, 27, 44–51, 57,
66–67, 103, 124–126, 128, 158, 164–166,
170, 211–212; of adults 45, 164;
providing activities 48; supportive
services for 45
care homes 127, 154; pandemic 154
CARES Act 64, 127

Centers for Disease Control and Prevention
(CDC) 25–26, 43–44, 63–64, 69–70, 74, 81,
87–88, 105–106, 114, 119–120, 124, 225
Chen, Jarvis 10
children 11, 18, 36–37, 44–45, 51, 71, 126–127,
197, 215
Chonody, J. 25
chronic diseases 74, 106–107, 157, 198
cognitive impairments 211
community-based services 135, 141, 153
community care 78, 123, 125, 145–146; policy
initiative 146
community practice 141–143
community stakeholders 37
comorbidities 11, 110–111, 148, 154, 201
competing responsibilities 51
coronavirus disease (COVID-19) 2–3, 9–19,
43–47, 49–51, 57–60, 63–67, 78–79, 87–89,
92–102, 104–107, 109–111, 118–122,
124–128, 135–142, 148–150, 179–204,
213–230, 232–236, 239–241, 243–244;
infection 10, 201, 204–205; nursing home
social work during 161; and older adults 75;
outbreak 20, 43, 49–50, 96, 154, 156, 161,
196, 232–233, 236; outcomes 105–107; racism
96–97
Council on Social Work Education (CSWE)
27–28, 57, 70, 75, 97, 143
cultural geriatric mental health-care 175

Deaf older adults (DOA) 105–107
Dell, N. A. 169
dementia 27, 45, 47, 88, 97, 121, 124–125, 128,
145, 148–150, 193
Detroit's efforts 221
developmental disabilties 102
digital divide 26, 184
digital world 187–188
DiMaggio, P. 188
direct care workers 79, 170
disparities 17–18, 21, 35–36, 38, 64, 67, 114–116,
118, 120, 123, 127
Drum, C. E. 106

East Asian older adults 96
emergency management 157
essential items, delivery of 48
essential workers 38, 78, 122, 149
ethnicity 35, 57, 119, 121, 127
ethnic minority older adults 87

face masks 38, 106–107, 230, 233
family caregivers 44–45, 47–49, 51, 126, 139, 172
family caregiving 16, 44
FamilyMeans 46
family members 45, 48, 50–51, 57, 65, 69–70, 99, 103–104, 148–149, 161, 165, 192, 234
Farmer, P. 225
fear 36, 38, 87–88, 114–115, 149, 152–153, 161–162, 165, 169, 201–202, 204, 230, 233–236
financial capability 59
formal healthcare 235–236

gerontological social work 2–4, 14, 16–19, 21, 25–29, 32, 36–38, 57–58, 60, 63, 66–67, 81, 209–211
gerontological social workers (GSWs) 81–82, 93–94
gerontology-curriculum 74
Ghana 181, 201–202, 204, 214–215, 233–235, 243–244
Gilbert, M. 202
global pandemic 44, 51–52, 114, 193, 195; *see also* coronavirus disease (COVID-19)
goal-directed wellness plans 218
grandchildren 36, 48, 126–127
grandparent caregivers 126
grandparents 16, 37, 126–128
Gyasi, R. M. 234–235

Hakim, D. 102
healthcare 9–10, 17–18, 78–79, 100, 110, 115, 118, 198, 204, 232–233, 235–236, 244; providers 106–107; services 20, 107, 139, 244; systems 78, 80, 233, 243–244
health facilities 235–236
health gap 58, 66
Healthier Black Elders Center (HBEC) 229
health literacy 105
health-seeking behavior 233, 236
health workers 234–236
heightened inequality 63–64
home and community-based services (HCBS) 135; self-direction of 135
home care 122–123, 139, 146; services 122, 139
home health care workers 78–80
Human Immunodeficiency Virus (HIV) 81, 109–111; care 109–111; treatment outcomes 109

immigrants 34, 99–100
inaccessible COVID-19 testing 107

inaccessible public information 106
influenza pandemic 81
informal caregiving 47
Innovative Telephone Outreach Program 228
Inslee, Jay 10
instrumental support 165–166, 210
intellectual disabilties 102
intergenerational solidarity 20–21
internal conflict 201
interprofessional practice 26–27
intersectionality 17–18, 21, 57, 121

Jones, C. 212
Jones, V. Nikki 10
Journal of Gerontological Social Work (JGSW) 2, 10, 58, 60

Kaiser Family Foundation 43, 110, 119, 121
Kerson, T. S. 81
kinship care 126
Korea Centers for Disease Control and Prevention [KCDC] 145
Kornfeld-Matte, Rosa 127
Krieger, Nancy 10
Kushalnagar, P. 105
Kusmaul, N. 209–210

Latinx 10, 92, 99–100
leadership 59–60, 143
legally responsible relatives 137
LGBTQ 114–116
LGBTQA+ older adults 87
lifestyle leaders 209–210
Lightfoot, E. 125
living facilities 43, 45, 69, 71, 74
lockdown 149, 195, 201–202, 214
loneliness 19, 26–27, 65–66, 87–88, 119, 121–122, 169, 173, 175–176, 192–194, 209, 211, 215, 217, 228–229
long-term care facilities 43–44, 48–51, 64, 106, 135, 152–153, 182, 211
long-term HIV survivors 110–111
low-and middle-income countries (LMICs) 175, 214, 232–236
low socioeconomic status 71, 88

mental health care 172, 176, 221
mental health services 71, 97
mental illness 164–166, 169
minority groups 87, 119
Moore, T. 125
moral panic 202
Morrow-Howell, N. 35
multi-sectoral synergies 202

National Association of Social Workers 57, 69–70, 74, 82, 88
National Digital Inclusion Alliance 228

Nigeria 148–150, 233–234
nursing facilities 69, 135, 138, 152, 161
nursing home care 122, 124
nursing homes 11, 15, 17–18, 43–45, 59–60, 74, 120, 122, 124, 149, 152–153, 156–158, 161–162
nursing home social work 161

older adults: advanced home care for 139; chat robot for 211; COVID-19 and 74–75; digital exclusion of 187; with disabilities 65, 88; healthcare concerns of 232, 235; in poverty 64; re-integrating 204
older adults with hearing loss (OAHL) 105–107
older adults with serious mental illnesses (OASMI) 169–170
older Black adults 192–193
older latinx immigrants 99
older people, social responses for 195
older workers: in aging America 32; within Senior Community Service Employment Program 33
on-line connection, service provision 20
online informal support 50
othering language 11

Parnett, W. E. 82
Peprah, P. 235
physical distancing 79, 93, 181–182, 187–192, 209–210, 228
positive religious coping 193
poverty 35, 63–66, 69, 87–88, 111, 118, 120–121, 126–128, 185, 240
psychosocial challenges 110
psychosocial effects 109
psychosocial support 148–150
public health emergencies 96, 156, 201
Puerto Rico 224–225

quality of care, monitor 49

race 10, 12, 17, 35, 57, 87, 118–121, 127–128
racial group 87
Rauktis, M. E. 218
reduced patronage 243
resilience 116, 156, 209, 230
risk factors 10, 26, 102, 106, 116, 120–121, 148, 191, 209, 217
Rothstein, M. A. 82

Sands, L. P. 225
SARs 63, 82, 156, 211
SDH framework 63–67
self-directed budgets 137
self-direction 135–138
self-direction model 136
Senior Community Service Employment Program (SCSEP) 31–38, 59

serious mental illness 169
service enrollment 89
SGL elders 114–115
social care 2–3, 172, 176, 192–193, 240–241
social distancing 44–45, 87, 105, 114–115, 124–125, 149, 152, 181, 190, 192, 215, 218, 226, 228
social exclusion 89, 187–188
social isolation 2–3, 19, 26–27, 48, 59–60, 65–67, 87–89, 110, 115, 121–122, 128, 176, 181–182, 192–194, 217, 221–222, 228–229
social justice 14, 57, 70, 118, 184
social networks 19, 121, 188, 192, 214–215, 234
social protection agencies 214–215, 236
social security schemes, in Ghana 214
social support networks 176, 214–215, 234
social work 2–3, 18, 21, 25–29, 31, 57–60, 65–66, 69, 103–104, 127, 129, 161–162, 230, 232; education 3, 27–28, 57, 60, 75, 97, 128, 204; grand challenges for 58, 65–66; practice 2–3, 118, 193, 219, 224; programs 28, 74–75, 97; responses 81, 102, 217; scholars 2, 26, 32, 35–38; values 69–70, 80
social workers (SWs) 14–21, 25–26, 66–67, 69–71, 74–75, 78–79, 81–82, 92–93, 96–97, 102–105, 120–128, 141–142, 149–150, 161–162, 164–166, 172–173, 184–185, 193, 209–210, 217–219
South Korea 145, 211
special needs groups 124
spirituality 94, 193
staying isolated, stay safe 209
stigmatization 82, 125, 204–205
strength-based perspective 15, 18, 21
Sunshine 211–212
systems-level change 142

technological support 123
transmission risk 79, 146

United Nations Development Program (UNDP) 232
United States' Substance Abuse and Mental Health Services Administration 170

Vietnam 63, 195–197, 199
virtual engagement 89
virtual social work care 192–193
vulnerable populations 66, 88, 111, 166, 182, 204, 222, 226

Wang, D. 25
workers 11, 16, 21, 31–34, 37–38, 44, 48–49, 59, 64, 67, 78–79, 135–136
World Bank 239–240
World Health Organization (WHO) 63, 96, 99, 114, 148–149, 156, 195, 201–202, 204, 233, 239–240

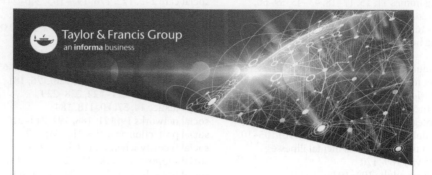